Feed Your Kids Well

Feed Your Kids Well

How to Help Your Child
Lose Weight and Get Healthy

Fred Pescatore, M.D., M.P.H.

John Wiley & Sons, Inc.

New York • Chichester • Weinheim • Brisbane • Singapore • Toronto

Copyright © 1998 by Fred Pescatore. All rights reserved
Published by John Wiley & Sons, Inc.
Published simultaneously in Canada

The information contained in this book is not intended to serve as a replacement for professional medical advice. Any use of the information in this book is at the reader's discretion. The author and publisher specifically disclaim any and all liability arising directly or indirectly from the use or application of any information contained in this book. A health care professional should be consulted regarding your specific situation.

Library of Congress Cataloging-in-Publication Data:
Pescatore, Fred
Feed your kids well: how to help your child lose weight and get healthy /
Fred Pescatore.
p. cm.
Includes index.
ISBN 0-471-24855-X (hardcover: alk. paper)
1. Obesity in children—Treatment. 2. Reducing diets.
3. Children—Nutrition. I. Title.
RJ399.C6P47 1998
613.2'083—dc21
                                                                98-13103

Printed in the United States of America

10 9 8 7 6 5 4 3 2 1

Author's Note

The information in this book reflects the author's experience and is not intended to replace the advice of your pediatrician. It is not the intent of the author to diagnose or prescribe treatment. The intent is only to help your child gain health and lose weight, in conjunction with the cooperation of your child's pediatrician. Only your pediatrician can determine if this nutritional lifestyle plan is suitable for your child. In addition to regular checkups and supervision, any questions or symptoms that may arise should be addressed to your child's pediatrician.

This book is not meant to serve as a replacement for your pediatrician. Rather, it should be used as an adjunct or an alternative to what you've been hearing for many years on what to feed your children. The dietary recommendations in this book are for all children, not just for those who are overweight.

In the event you use this information without your doctor's approval, you are prescribing for yourself, and the publisher and the author assume no responsibility.

This book is dedicated to SHF, whose
inspiration made this possible

Contents

ACKNOWLEDGMENTS   xi

FOREWORD BY ROBERT C. ATKINS, M.D.   xiii

INTRODUCTION   1

PART ONE: UNDERSTANDING THE BASICS OF BETTER HEALTH   7
  1 A Personal Story   9
  2 The Obesity Epidemic   13
  3 Weight, Metabolism, and Self-esteem   21
  4 Sugar Blues   31
  5 The Great Fat Myth   50
  6 Carbohydrates—Separating Fact from Hype   65

PART TWO: THE NEXT GENERATION DIET   73
  7 Pre-Diet Instruction Manual   75
  8 Unlocking the Mysteries of the Diet   82
  9 The New Pyramid Effect   88
 10 The Next Generation Diet, Phase 1:
    Weight Loss for Children of All Ages   92
 11 The Next Generation Diet: Ages 6–8   104
 12 The Next Generation Diet: Ages 9–12   109
 13 The Next Generation Diet: Teenagers   113
 14 The Next Generation Diet, Phase 2 :
    The Healthy Step—The General Rules   117
 15 The Next Generation Diet, Phase 3 :
    A Lifetime of Healthy Eating   122
 16 How to Make the Diet Even More Successful   127

PART THREE: THE HEALTH CONNECTION: HOW TO PREVENT DISEASE   135
 17 Your Child's Health   137
 18 The Insulin Factor and Diabetes   143
 19 Syndrome X   148

20 The Great Cholesterol Debate ... 153

21 Yeast Inflates More Than Bread ... 162

22 Allergies and Food Sensitivities ... 175

23 Asthma ... 180

24 The Common Cold, Earaches, and Other Complaints ... 186

25 Attention Deficit Disorder and Attention
Deficit Hyperactivity Disorder ... 191

26 Nutrients and Supplements ... 199

27 Shaping the Future ... 208

PART FOUR: THE HEALTHY FITNESS ZONE ... 221

28 Couch Potatoes Start as Little Spuds ... 223

29 Demystifying Exercise ... 231

PART FIVE: MEAL PLANS AND RECIPES ... 241

30 Sample Menu Selections ... 243

31 Recipes ... 255

REFERENCES ... 279

INDEX ... 285

Acknowledgments

There are many people who helped along the way in this labor of love and who deserve to be acknowledged:

JW and LW for starting the whole process
LC for keeping a secret and for her support
EM for believing this could happen
KP for taking all my phone calls
HC, GM, PM, EI and JB for being them
MCR for her great recipe suggestions
WO for teaching me about computers
KP, JE and JE for putting up with me
RCA for being a mentor and a friend
FG for being a great nutritionist and friend
My parents for the ultimate inspiration
TM, my editor, for putting the book together so well
CS for his great work, understanding, patience, and perseverance
And lastly to all my patients, young and old alike, for being a constant source of inspiration and pleasure for me.

I thank you all.

Foreword
by Robert C. Atkins, M.D.

I'm very happy to be writing the Foreword to this book. For years, I've been treating adults with nutritional medicine with overwhelming success. But why wait until you're an adult to feed yourself well? It makes all the sense in the world to start a healthier way of being in childhood.

Our children are having more problems than ever before. You might find it interesting to revisit your old sixth-grade classroom. Remember how few of your classmates were overweight? Well, look at their successors now. I'll bet you'll note a mini-epidemic of overweight children.

That's just the visible side of the problem. Delve further and you may find that two in every ten schoolchildren have been prescribed the stimulant drug Ritalin because their hyperactivity or inconstant attention spans make the teachers' problems too difficult.

Type II diabetes, something that heretofore required a minimum of three decades to develop, is beginning to be seen in high school students.

The sad news is that all of these problems are obvious consequences of a culturewide series of nutritional mistakes. Yet the leaders of medicine are not only perplexed by the epidemic nature of these and similar problems, they continue to perpetuate the same mistakes that have caused these problems.

Many are the hours that my practice associate, Dr. Fred Pescatore, the Associate Medical Director of the Atkins Center for Complementary Medicine, has talked with me about the vast gulf between the successful results our school-age patients were getting and the lack of success their previous medical management had provided. We agreed that the failure to recognize the harmful consequences of repeated courses of antibiotics or of constantly recycling environmental chemicals created many of their problems, but we were amazed by mainstream medicine's utter failure to recognize the harmful effects on our children's health of junk food containing the refined carbohydrates—sugars and starches. And we wondered when they would realize that their insistence on restricting fats has only led to an increasing intake of junk carbohydrates. That advice has only been part of the problem, not its solution.

Feed Your Kids Well provides that solution. It is based not only on an understanding of what children must learn to eat and to avoid in order to maintain ideal health, but also on targeting of vitanutrient intake to correct the medical crises our children face.

The information in *Feed Your Kids Well* is accessible and has been time-tested by the Atkins Center medical staff. You'll find that its suggestions make sense. The most pleasant surprise of all is that the food and nutrition plans Dr. Pescatore suggests will be accepted by most children because the often-immediate improvements they will feel can prove to be self-motivating.

Feed Your Kids Well contains a message that all parents need to learn—junk food and pharmaceuticals both have significant downside risks. If we get our children to avoid both of them, we can allow them to thrive in ideal health.

Dr. Pescatore teaches you, step by step, just how easy and rewarding that can be.

Introduction
by Fred Pescatore, M.D.

A refrain I hear over and over from the children who come to see me is, "I wanna be healthy." They wanna be healthy but don't know how. And how could they? They are children, and what they know is what they learn from their parents, teachers, and other children. But they can be healthy. This book is the tool that concerned parents can use to help their overweight and nonoverweight children get healthy.

I am living proof that health is an attainable goal. I was an overweight child. If you've never struggled with a weight problem, it's a condition to which you will never quite be able to relate. Being fat distorts your body perception, gives you a poor self-image, and often leaves you open to ridicule.

That's only what being overweight can do to your child when he or she is young. There are lifelong psychological and physical implications. No matter how slender I might be today, inside there will always be that overweight little boy, longing to be thin and athletic, to fit in. Today, I am exactly the right weight for my size, but I still carry the baggage that will, I'm sure, remain with me for the rest of my life.

I wish my parents had *Feed Your Kids Well* when they were raising me. Over the years, I have spent a good deal of time undoing the many harmful (albeit well-meaning) eating habits they instilled in me. It's important to understand that habits are all they are. Proper eating, like proper manners and grooming, must be taught. Too often, parents don't realize this.

I host a weekly radio show. When I interview an author, one of the first questions I ask is how he or she came to write; the answer tells me a good deal about the person. I'd like to share with you some of my background and how it affected who I am today and why I'm writing this book.

My quest for knowledge has taken me all over the globe to look for the most beneficial ways of treating my patients. I tell my patients that I will do almost anything that will make them well. That is my job, and I take it seriously.

Even as a child I knew I wanted to be a physician. There was never any other consideration for me. I wanted to help other people—and myself. During my medical training in New York City, I was exposed to the latest scientific breakthroughs. I was trained in a completely conventional (allopathic) medical way, and I would have been satisfied with that approach—if only the majority of the patients I saw were getting better. That wasn't the case and it concerned me. I began to think that there must be something else that could be done, that there had to be more to healing than what we were doing in the hospital. I wasn't naive enough to think everyone should live forever, but I was idealistic enough to believe we could be doing more for our patients.

Fortunately, right after residency training, I stumbled upon complementary medicine, a completely new concept for me. Complementary medicine involves looking for the source of a person's medical complaint, not just attacking symptoms. Complementary medicine challenges the physician to find the answer and the cure. It involves using alternative medical techniques along with those learned in traditional medical schools.

I have been fortunate to train with one of the founding fathers of complementary medicine, Dr. Robert Atkins. Many of you know him as "the diet doctor," but he's much more than that. He has been treating patients in a complementary fashion for more than thirty years. I was able to draw on his experience and to develop my own ideas on nutrition and vitamin supplementation, allowing me to offer patients more than just one drug after another.

Feed Your Kids Well comes at a time when the medical establishment is finally beginning to realize that alternative treatments exist and are flourishing. In the past year, over one in three Americans visited an alternative medical practitioner, and yet there have not been many doctors discussing the benefits of alternative medical techniques for our children. If you are comfortable exploring alternative techniques for yourself—and you've found success with them—the next logical step would be for your children to share in that success.

Through my years working with Dr. Atkins, I developed my own ideas about health and nutrition, and I have put these ideas to the test with my patients. Some of Dr. Atkins's ideas and mine are similar, while some of them are quite different. His very successful weight-loss diet involves achieving a metabolic state called *ketosis*, which occurs when the body is actively metabolizing stored fat. Because children are more metabolically active than adults, my nutrition plan, the *Next Generation Diet*, does not call for your child to achieve this state. I'd like to believe I've taken Dr. Atkins's work to the next level—the next generation.

Feed Your Kids Well includes a nutritional lifestyle program that incorporates the important building blocks—protein, fats, and carbohydrates—combining them in a complete, well-balanced meal plan that is easy to maintain over a lifetime. Part One of the book explains the science behind your child's body and metabolism. The diet outlined in Part Two will enable your overweight child to lose weight and to become more healthy. Part Three explores the treatment of some of the most common childhood illnesses in ways your child's pediatrician may not have told you about. It also explores many other diet-related illnesses to which your child may be unknowingly susceptible because of his or her diet.

These principles apply to all children—overweight or not. Part Four covers the role of exercise. My program is linked to an exercise plan to ensure success. Exercise has become almost anathema to many of our children; each year, less and less time is spent in the pursuit of physical activity. I will discuss the importance of exercise and many ways you can incorporate this into your and your family's daily routine. In Part Five, I offer sugar-free menu and recipe sections that will enable you to make great meals that have withstood life's toughest critics—children and teenagers.

The beauty of The Next Generation Diet is its simplicity. You need not concern yourself with calorie counts or monitor the fat intake. The diet does this for you automatically. Calories don't count, and your child will never go hungry. The *only* thing you have to monitor is the number of grams of carbohydrates that are present in the foods you feed your child. I'll teach you how to do just that. This information is contained on the nutrition label located on the packaging of most foods. To make it easier, I often recommend that my patients buy an inexpensive companion carbohydrate counter they can use to help them plan each meal.

Part of treating a patient in an integrative way involves the use of oral nutritional supplementation—taking vitamins, minerals, and sometimes herbal preparations. I contend that it is possible to treat many common childhood illnesses without the use of harmful drugs. I'll share some of my time-tested favorite supplements with you throughout this book. At the very least, these nutritional supplements may be used in combination with drugs your pediatrician has recommended in order to achieve the optimal health picture for your child. It's important for you to understand that I do not mean for this book to be a replacement for your child's pediatrician, who is very important to the well-being of your child. I simply offer additional advice that has worked in the hundreds of children I've treated.

I believe we are at a health crisis point. Never before have there been so many overweight adults and so many overweight children. What is being overweight? It's partly based on a scientific ratio that I'll explain to you, and it's partly based on social norms. I'll provide you ways to determine if your own kid is overweight.

According to the National Health and Nutrition Exam Survey, approximately 26 percent, or one in four, of all American children and adolescents are overweight. That is double the rate of thirty years ago. Between 1963 and today, this rate has increased by 54 percent among children aged six to eleven and thirty-nine percent among adolescents aged twelve to eighteen. In the case of a child, obesity, as opposed to simply being overweight, is defined as being greater than 130 percent of the ideal body weight for the child's height. Using these figures, 14 percent of all children and 12 percent of adolescents are obese. When the figures for overweight and obese children are combined, we find that nearly one in three children has a weight problem, while half of all adults are overweight. You can see that this problem is of epidemic proportions—an epidemic that has occurred despite the years of what I call the "low-fat myth." The low-fat, high-carbohydrate diet was proposed as the ultimate healthy diet because in the athletes who ate this way, cholesterol levels and other health indicators were favorable. However, because most Americans are sedentary and not at all athletic, I feel that advocating this diet has been a great disservice to the American people.

All current indicators show that the health of the American population—adults and children—has gotten worse, not better, since the low-fat diet has become the standard. Even if the low-fat diet is okay for some people, it clearly is not the diet for the majority of the population. Instead of eating meat, people now pile their plates with pasta and think they are eating wisely. In this book I will show you how this is equivalent to piling your plate with sugar. It is my contention that the interaction of sugar and carbohydrates with proteins and fats—not just fat alone or genetics—has led to this obesity epidemic in our children.

As I researched this book, I was amazed to find that there was no similar book that portrays sugar as the "food criminal" for children. This is odd because there have been many diets for adults that view sugar this way. By far the most famous and successful is the phenomenal bestseller *Dr. Atkins' New Diet Revolution.*

Being overweight is far more than just a cosmetic problem, although it's sometimes treated that way. It can be the cause of a host of health-related problems. Only now, after years of research, are we beginning to realize that the preventable harm we cause our bodies when we are young takes its toll on us as adults. Furthermore, because obesity is affecting a younger and younger segment of the population, diseases—diabetes, heart disease, hypertension, sleep apnea, orthopedic abnormalities, and others—once confined to adults are now becoming increasingly prevalent in our youth. If we don't do something to stop the obesity epidemic, the next generation could suffer these horrible and potentially fatal diseases as regularly as we suffered from chicken pox when we were young.

My original purpose for this book was to provide a weight-loss book for children. However, as I thought about it over the period of several months, it became clearer to me that through a healthy diet many childhood illnesses, including allergies, asthma, and even attention deficit disorder, could be tempered and brought under control without the use of potentially harmful medications, which in fact, might even be a cause of these illnesses.

Don't kid yourself, it's not just baby fat, and it's not just big bones. I can't tell you how many times I've heard those excuses, offered by overprotective parents and grandparents to spare themselves pain. I say this because parents must often make difficult adjustments in their own lives and their own eating habits in order to make successful changes for their children.

No matter how precocious your child may be, it is important to remember that he or she is not merely a pint-sized version of an adult. Some parents forget this and believe that they can simply place their overweight child on a diet designed for an adult. Be forewarned: an adult dietary plan cannot be used for any of your children, overweight or not. Chances are that not only won't the adult diet work, but it could conceivably do damage to healthy growth patterns and the normal maturation of your child.

An adult diet is no more suitable for a child than is a television program or movie that has been designed specifically for mature audiences. Children require different nutritional balances at different stages of their lives. For this reason it is not practical or healthy to put your overweight child—or any child—on any of the numerous adult diets.

Stop to think about it for a moment. It would be inconceivable for a parent to feed an infant anything but food especially formulated for them. Yet, once the child is able to speak and eat on his or her own, this same parent wouldn't think twice about giving their toddler or preschooler exactly what they themselves would eat or exactly what the child wants to eat. Suddenly, nutrition takes a back seat to everything else.

This book will help you avoid those mistakes by giving you hints on how to handle even the most stress-inducing children in their pursuit of proper eating habits. I discuss children who have terrible eating habits, like those who choose to eat only junk food or those who won't sit at the table with the family.

The earlier in life you start any program, the greater is the chance of a lifetime of success, and it is possible to start a diet protocol for any child starting at the age of two. I encourage dietary modifications for the children of my patients this young, but I won't be offering that advice in this book. This is a highly individualized segment of the pediatric population, and I would feel uncomfortable offering advice where I could not personally oversee the results. This book is therefore designed for kids from ages six to eighteen.

Feed Your Kids Well is divided into sections devoted to specific age groups. Please keep in mind that these age groups are only suggestions. For example, a very large five-year-old can certainly be started on the diet. A small thirteen-year-old may fit better in the nine to twelve category than in the teenage one. No one knows your child better than you, and common sense in this regard should prevail when deciding in which age group to place your child.

The inspiration for this work comes from my patients, a constant source of enjoyment and encouragement to me. I've successfully treated and helped hundreds of children and thousands of adult patients lose weight and attain health. It is extremely rewarding to me to offer a program that enriches the lives of so many people. It was at my patients' prompting that I ultimately agreed to share this nutritional plan with the rest of the world. It is my strongest desire that the next generation of children do not have to grow up the way I did.

Many of the success stories you will read are about the children of my adult patients. These parents were so unhappy with the treatment their children were getting from their regular pediatricians (in many cases, it was simply a matter of drug after drug) that they brought them to me, knowing from their own experience that their children would get well and flourish. Each story you will read about in this book is true. The name of each patient has been changed to protect his or her privacy.

My ultimate aim is to offer a comprehensive nutritional lifestyle plan that can and will work not only for your child, but for the entire family. You can't isolate one child from siblings, adults in the household, or the outside world. Parents cannot do this important work alone; your children are being minded by many people other than you. Anyone who takes an active caregiver role for your child also needs to read this book. This especially means anyone doing the grocery shopping and meal preparation. This will probably include siblings, grandparents, or household help.

The plan I'm outlining will work not only in the initial phases when everyone is enthusiastic about it, but also in the more difficult maintenance phases when the program needs to be reinforced in order to guarantee a lifetime of healthy eating. Once the honeymoon phase of the diet is over and the real work begins, it is a supportive family that will ensure the longest lasting effects.

I hope *Feed Your Kids Well* will help you instill in your children a sense of responsibility for one's own actions, including making the correct decisions about what to eat. They need to learn that a healthy diet-and-exercise program will enhance every aspect of their lives.

So do something about your children's weight if they are overweight, and if they are not, do something about their diet in order to prevent them from becoming victims of a diet-related illness. One of my goals is to make you think twice about what you feed your entire family, including yourself. If you feed your kids well, you can help ensure a lifetime of good health for your children—the best legacy of all.

PART ONE

Understanding *the* Basics *of* Better Health

A Personal Story

I GREW UP IN WHAT WE CONSIDERED TO BE A TYPICAL ITALIAN-AMERICAN family. Everyone was obese—my mother, my father, and my two sisters. It wasn't even a topic for conversation because, to us, it was the norm. Italians ate. We ate. And we ate a lot. So what?

The mainstay at each meal was pasta. Pasta and bread, followed by a course of meat. No matter what the main course was, we would start with pasta. And there was no such thing as eating *only* everything on your plate. In our household, if you didn't ask for seconds, then there had to be something wrong with you. If you didn't eat enough, you were probably coming down with something that might require a doctor's attention.

Naturally, because this was my only dining experience, I thought this was the way everybody ate. In fact, when I visited other people's homes and saw that they didn't eat that way, I thought they were odd, that they were the ones who were out of step with the rest of the world. Where was the pasta course? Something was terribly wrong. Didn't they know what a real meal was? I would often come home hungry and my mother would feed me again, only this time what she considered a proper dinner. I was even encouraged not to go out to eat because the food wouldn't be very good and I'd come home hungry.

the weight issue

Was weight an issue in our family? Absolutely not. After all, coming from a tight-knit family, we thought everybody lived and ate like we did. There was no standard to compare ourselves to, other than us. Should weight have been an issue in our family? You better believe it! I was overweight, as were my two older sisters. Both my parents were also overweight. The sad thing was, because my parents did not see this as a problem, neither did any of their children. Sure, my sisters attempted to lose weight every so often, but because there was no support from my parents, who were always pushing food in front of us, they were doomed to failure. And, as a result, they still are overweight. Neither of them has ever been able to maintain weight loss from the numerous diets they've tried over the years. Perhaps I was more fortunate in my attempt to lose weight because I had the advantage of being the youngest child. I was able to see the way my sisters were constantly sabotaged, and I knew that when I did make the attempt, I had to do it without the prior knowledge and consent of my parents and without listening to their advice and recommendations.

This is not to say that I don't love my parents or value their advice about other issues. It's just that they didn't have the knowledge to handle this problem. They were great parents in every other way and provided me with the means to achieve as much as I have. I just wish they had had this book to help guide them when I was growing up.

By the time I was fifteen years old, I was five feet ten inches tall and weighed a whopping 240 pounds! My life was a mess. I suffered from asthma and various allergies. I couldn't play sports because I didn't have the stamina. The truth was I could hardly move. Socially I was an outcast. I was teased unmercifully by my peers, which caused me to be deeply ashamed of my obesity and, by extension, myself.

As you can imagine, I was desperately unhappy. I wanted to do what my friends were doing. I wanted to play singles on the tennis team, but I just didn't have the endurance. Finally, I was so miserable that I realized I had to do something. It was Lent, the forty-day period of time when Christians will forgo eating food they like or participating in activities they enjoy in order to commemorate Jesus spending forty days in the desert without food and water. So I made a secret deal with myself that for forty days and forty nights I would give up all solid food.

Without any supervision or guidance whatsoever, I embarked upon a crash starvation diet. I drank diet soda and nothing else. By the end of forty days and forty nights, I had lost sixty pounds. But it was not without paying a steep price. Before beginning the diet, I was a straight A student. By the time it ended, I could hardly pay attention in class and my grades had plummeted. My stomach shrank, which was a perfect setup for a lifetime of yo-yo dieting. My body started to break down, and I began to lose muscle tissue. I was sixty pounds lighter, but my body and mind were suffering potentially dire consequences. At this point, as you might well imagine, my mother was beside herself. There were constant fights and attempts at bribery to get me to resume eating "regularly." My parents thought there was something wrong with me and even went so far as to take me to see several physicians and priests. But to no avail. At this point, I was finally going to take control of my life and see my way to a skinnier me.

revelation: losing weight means getting healthier

In spite of my poor dietary habits, I had managed to lose an enormous amount of weight, and by the time I was finished with my crash diet, I found there was an added bonus: my allergies and asthma had amazingly disappeared. Once I began on my own version of a maintenance diet, which consisted primarily of meats and salads, my stamina returned and my mind cleared. Without realizing it, by losing weight and changing the foods I ate, I had become a healthier person. For the first time in my life, I began to equate what I ate with how I felt. It was only after this experience that it occurred to me that proper eating should be as ingrained in our psyches as is washing our hands before eating and brushing our teeth after meals. I only wish I'd had that knowledge long before I became an obese teenager. It was such a simple lesson to learn: What you place into your body becomes a part of you and can affect how you feel!

If I had grown up with this knowledge as simply another part of the value system my parents had instilled in me, I would never have become obese, and my whole life would not be centered around the struggle with weight as it is today.

I had lost the weight, but as anyone who has a weight problem knows, that's only half the battle. I had to keep the weight off. And, to this day, the maintenance of this weight loss remains a problem.

Since the time of my initial weight loss, I have been on numerous fad diets, many of which I've made up myself. Some of the more humorous ones include the french fry/chocolate pudding diet I was fond of in medical school. Another diet I was partial to in medical school was the egg white/spinach diet. I should mention that somehow I managed to lose weight on both these diets, but do either of these sound particularly healthy to you? Of course not. The truth is, because of a young person's metabolism, he or she will be able to lose weight on most any diet, but the results won't necessarily be healthy.

Even now, twenty years after I lost all that weight, I still think about food pretty much constantly throughout the day. Perhaps this can be somewhat explained by the fact that I practice nutritional medicine, but I think there's more to it than that. At this point, it is relatively easy for me to know what it is I can and cannot eat, but at times I have to be stricter with myself than at other times.

Your children can avoid these troubles. You need only arm them with the necessary nutritional information and then consider it important enough to work with your children to stick to healthy eating. It is my goal that this book help you do just this: Give your child the legacy of good eating habits—and a trim, healthy body.

The Obesity
Epidemic

it can't happen to *my* child

Youngsters care about being overweight. I know of one six-year-old girl who, overly concerned about her weight (in truth, she was, at most, just a few pounds overweight), put herself on what amounted to a starvation diet. She refused to eat any solid food at all and would drink only juice, and that sparingly. Eventually, the situation became so serious that her parents needed to put her in the hospital, where she was fed intravenously. At the same time, she was put into counseling to help her deal with her skewed self-image. Finally, after months of therapy, she finally consented to eating solid food. Nevertheless, to this day she is exceedingly vigilant as to her weight. And remember, this is a mere *six-year-old!*

adjusting our attitudes

Not long ago, a patient with a weight problem visited my office. As she removed her coat, she remarked casually, "My nephew was at a birthday party the other day, and they served pizza, cake, and ice cream. You know—all the *good* stuff." She paused a moment, then sighed with envy, "Isn't it great that kids can get away with eating like that? I sure wish I could eat that way and not gain weight."

This attitude toward children and food reveals a terrible misconception that has led to millions of American children being overweight. And perhaps even more importantly, these same children, their eating patterns established early in life, grow up to be adults who are constantly battling a weight problem, which inevitably dooms them to a lifelong struggle against obesity.

As parents, we are generally aware that the habits, values, and disciplines we instill in our children will serve them throughout their lives. Yet, oddly enough we cling to the misguided notion that in terms of their eating habits, children are a species apart from the rest of the human race, that commonsense rules and well-established laws of cause and effect do not apply.

There is an old maxim that goes, "Give me a child for the first seven years, and you may do what you like with him afterwards." The seeds of what become our personalities, our likes, our dislikes, and even our eating habits are sown early. Show me the food intake of a child, and I will show you the dietary and health problems that child will have as an adult. The nutritional lifestyle program I offer you in this book will help all children get healthy, not just those who are overweight.

American culture has spread its tentacles across the planet and, unfortunately, even our bad eating habits are mirrored in emerging cultures. Countries that newly experience economic wealth inevitably change their eating habits to the point where more sugar and refined carbohydrates are ingested.

In this country, we are faced with an obesity epidemic that unquestionably begins in childhood. Some nutrition experts have even gone so far as to call ours a "fat enabling" culture. Examples abound: the colossal buckets of buttered popcorn now standard at movie theaters, the half-gallon of soda that has become an accepted serving size, the half-pound cinnamon bun served at every mall across America, the growing sizes of restaurant portions.

And let us not forget America's fascination for and craving of anything advertised as "low-fat," which a number of researchers have dubbed the "SnackWell phenomenon." The truth is, in the long run, not only is low-fat unhealthy for your child, but the overconsumption of any processed food product is ultimately damaging to his or her health. During processing, natural vitamins and minerals are taken out of the food. At best, they are replaced with chemical versions that the body cannot readily or completely absorb and thus are nutritionally useless. At worst, these natural nutrients are not replaced at all. The aim of the processors is to produce food more cheaply and with a longer shelf life, but the result is food that is not as healthy for us as it was originally. The plain fact is that these so-called low-fat health foods are not dietetic, and furthermore they are not even healthy.

Food producers and purveyors, well aware of our weaknesses, continually expand the choices and availability of such foods. Advertisers, who target impressionable children who tend to watch more television and attend more movies than adults, bombard us and our children with the not so subliminal message that it's okay to eat an entire box of cookies, so long as they are fat-free. Is it any wonder that our waistlines and the waistlines of our children are expanding at an alarming rate? It's too easy to be overweight in this country!

Yet most adults in this country seem to be perpetually concerned with their weight. If you have the slightest doubt, simply stop by your local bookstore and see how many diet tomes fill the shelves, or take notice of the thin, always-in-shape role models, both male and female, who peek out at us from the pages of fashion magazines or flash in front of us on virtually every television show and commercial. And how many households do you know of that don't have a bathroom scale or that go so far as to hide the scale away as if it is an evil entity?

the perils of "wonder drugs"

By the age of six, nearly 40 percent of American girls have expressed a desire to be thinner. By age nine, nearly 50 percent have dieted once and, by the age of sixteen, 45 percent will have put themselves on some kind of a crash diet. Even more disturbing is the fact that 15 percent take diet pills on a regular basis. Is this something you want for your child? I think not.

Between the time I wrote the first draft of this book and the time it went to print, there has been a recall and ban on two diet pills used in combination. We have witnessed the rise and fall of fen-phen, a drug combination that can cause a deadly heart-valve defect in many people, especially women.

There have been countless stories in the popular media and many more in the medical journals about children who have taken their lives or who have become addicted to medications in their quest for thinness.

Despite what new drug may come on the market between now and the time that you're reading this book, you can be certain that we will not know the long-term side effects. Furthermore, safety tests for new drugs are performed on adults and then the information is altered in a way so the doctor knows the dose for a child. Drug tests are not performed on children, and I would be loath to place my child on any medication until the long-term side effects had been studied in humans, not just laboratory test animals.

I think it's the wrong message to instill in our next generation that there's a pill for everything. Instead, we must instill a sense of responsibility for one's actions, even when it comes down to making the right decisions as to what to eat.

And if you're one of those who thinks I'm being an alarmist, I need only point out that thalidomide was considered a wonder drug until it was found to cause serious limb malformations in the fetuses of women who took the drug during pregnancy to avoid morning sickness. Wouldn't it be better if we were provided with all the necessary information about these drugs—not just the pros, but also the cons—before our children rely on them to handle their weight problem?

it's not just baby fat!

"Train up a child in the way he should go; and when he is old he will not depart from it."

—Proverbs XXII, 6

Some people are appalled by the idea of regulating a child's food intake. "He's so young. Why should I worry about what he eats now? He'll outgrow it, won't he?"

Nothing could be further from the truth. More often than not, children *won't* outgrow the eating patterns they set as children—they will have them for the rest of their lives. In fact, the older the obese child is, the greater the risk that obesity will continue into adulthood.

Consider these facts, compiled by the National Research Council:

41 percent of obese seven-year-olds become obese adults.

70 percent of obese ten-year-olds become obese adults.

And this pattern continues through adolescence. More than 80 percent of obese adolescents remain obese as adults. The severity of the obesity also factors into whether the obesity continues into adulthood. For instance, for those seven-year-olds who are 30 percent to 45 percent over their ideal weight, just half of these will be obese in adulthood. Among those same children who are 57 percent to 65 percent above their ideal weight, 80 percent, or four out of five, will be obese adults. And for those seven-year-olds who are over 65 percent of their ideal weight, virtually *all* will be obese.

It takes dedication and hard work to instill proper eating habits in children. But, in the end, they will appreciate it and so will you. I just wish my parents had had proper information as to how they should have been feeding me and my sisters.

Children don't have to be overweight. They can be taught early in life the proper way to eat. But until and unless parents understand that the roots of their child's eating problems start in childhood, their attempts at having their child lose weight are doomed to failure. By nature, parents want to give their children anything and everything to make them happy. But certainly this doesn't include anything that's bad for them or that will cause them discomfort, either now or in the future. For this reason, parents need to know what is good for their children to eat while making sure that it tastes good. At the same time, children need to know that making appropriate choices empowers them to do something positive about their weight.

Why are children in this country putting on so much excess weight? There are several reasons. For one thing, with the growing prevalence of the two-parent working household or the one-parent family, many youngsters frequently eat their meals away from home, without the guidance of a parent. Unfortunately, far too often this translates into reliance on the nutritional wasteland of fast food: candy, cookies, potato chips, pretzels, and other empty-calorie foods that can be grabbed easily on the run.

Although parents may believe that the nutritional situation is vastly improved if a child gets lunch at school, this is not always the case. Recent studies have shown that excess consumption of fruit juice leads to an increase in childhood obesity. It has been found that the average school-age boy drinks the equivalent of nearly three cans of soda a day, with girls' consumption close behind. They often get these beverages either in school or as part of a school lunch.

Professionals in the field of dietary needs are certainly aware of the problem and have tried to set guidelines. Unfortunately, these guidelines rarely work, primarily because most often they miss the mark. The National Cancer Institute has devised what they call "the five-a-day" program, which is designed to encourage people to eat five fruits and vegetables a day. Although this may be an optimistic figure, it is hoped that people will at least come close to this recommendation. Is this a realistic recommendation? Yes. Is this likely to happen, considering the way most kids eat today? Hardly, as you'll soon see for yourself.

fruit isn't all it's cracked up to be

In a study for her book, *Food Fight: A Guide to Eating Disorders for Pre-Teens and Their Parents*, author Janet Bode issued food diaries to eighty-seven students in three schools on Long Island and one in Brooklyn. The results were eye-opening. On the average, each child consumed 4.7 servings of fruits and vegetables (not including french fries) not a day, but a week! This translates into about half a serving a day, instead of the hoped-for five. And even more startling was that, of the eighty-seven students, seventeen ate no fruits or vegetables (except french fries). Often, when they did consume fruit, it was in the form of fruit juice, which lacks all-important fiber.

I think it is realistic to expect our children to eat their five a day, but I think it's more important for these five to come in the form of vegetables, rather than fruit. Fruit contains sugar, and by the end of this book, you'll know that the natural sugar found in fruit is the same as white sugar, which is the same as brown sugar, which is the same as many other hidden sugars.

I find that most parents don't like vegetables, therefore their children don't like them, so they are not a part of the meal. This is a serious problem. If we don't teach our children to appreciate vegetables at an early age, it will be increasingly difficult as they get older. We make sacrifices every day for our children, and eating vegetables should be something we're prepared to do.

When it comes to adding fruit to a child's diet, many well-meaning parents have leaped to the mistaken conclusion that substituting fruit juices for soda will help solve the problem. This is a dangerous misconception. After all, sugar behaves in the body the same way, no matter how it's delivered. So the fact that one beverage is filled with natural sugar and the other has added white cane sugar is of no difference and ultimately has the same effect on the nutritional status of your child.

Fruit juice is the dietary equivalent of drinking soda. As far as I'm concerned, there is absolutely no nutritional value in fruit juice. The vitamin C you can get from juice is too small an amount to compensate for all the sugar contained in that glass of juice. From a health standpoint, neither your overweight nor nonoverweight child should be drinking fruit juice because their body will have difficulty metabolizing all the sugar at once. This causes too much insulin to be secreted and may set your child up for a hypoglycemic reaction, among other things.

trick or treat?

All too often sweets are used as a reward. Who among us can't remember being coaxed by a parent to make an unpleasant visit, perhaps to a doctor or a dentist, with the promise that, "If you're good, we'll stop for ice cream on the way home." Maybe after visiting a doctor you were rewarded with a lollipop for good behavior. And what holiday, whether it be Christmas, Easter, Halloween, or Chanukah, isn't associated with chocolate, candy corn, or jelly beans? Is it any wonder then that sweetness equals reward, which translates into feeling good?

This, I feel, is a large part of the problem faced by overweight children and their well-meaning parents. And it's not only parents who unknowingly create roadblocks that prevent a child from eating properly. I've found that it is often grandparents or other caregivers who create some of these problems as well. With the increase in the number of children who are watched by people other than their parents—and this includes nannies, baby-sitters, and grandparents—it is necessary to explore that person's feeling concerning sugar, or we're setting up the program to fail.

the big bad wolf

Not long ago, I had a young couple bring in Steven, their four-year-old, who was experiencing behavioral problems at nursery school. The situation was so bad that Steven had been asked to leave three preschool programs because of these problems. Other tests showed that he also had several food sensitivities, which I will explain later. While I was reviewing all the laboratory data, his parents as well as his grandmother were present. I told the parents that Steven had to be taken off all sugar and simple carbohydrates. His parents were willing to try anything because they really wanted to handle this situation before their son had to go to elementary school. They were afraid he would carry the diagnosis of attention deficit hyperactivity disorder (ADHD, or ADD—the terms are often used interchangeably), which would place him in special education classes. This could be something that stigmatized the child for a lifetime.

Suddenly, his grandmother began to cry, not, I should say, because of these dire consequences. Instead, this woman was in tears because she felt as if I were trying to deprive her grandchild of something so special that removing these items from his diet would scar him more seriously than a diagnosis that would mean years of special education classes. After I was able to calm her down, I asked her if it was important to her that Steven felt well and was able to stay in school and perform well. She had to agree, though I'm sure she was still unconvinced that depriving Steven of sugar was the answer.

We need to look anywhere and everywhere we can if we are going to successfully raise a child with healthy eating habits. For each success, it becomes that much easier for an entire society to make these changes and for the entire population to become healthy.

Weight, Metabolism, and Self-esteem

"Mirror, Mirror on the Wall,
Who's the Fattest of Them All?"

THIS REFRAIN ACTUALLY WENT THROUGH MY HEAD AS A CHILD! I felt so hopeless about my situation that I began to conjure up outrageous images, as I peered tentatively toward and then away from my reflection in a full-length mirror. My self-esteem with regard to my appearance was really bad. I was lucky, though, because I had parents who never criticized my appearance—or the way I ate—and also because I was quite good in school. So there was some balance in my formative years.

But being overweight is far more than just a matter of cosmetics. It can and often does result in potentially serious physical and emotional problems, including grave social ramifications that can result in severe psychosocial stress. I should know. I was the kid who hated to go to school on gym days because I was afraid I would have to take my shirt off in front of the other students. I dreaded basketball season because of the inevitable Shirts vs. Skins competition, afraid that if I were to be chosen for the Skins team, I would have to take off my shirt, exposing myself to ridicule. And, even worse, what if I weren't chosen because of my enormous size? How embarrassing that would be!

I longed to be just like the rest of the kids, able to look into a mirror without flinching. But I knew that until I lost weight that would be impossible.

fat or pleasingly plump?

"I'm just a few pounds overweight. That's not so bad, is it?" is a common refrain I often hear. The truth is that it's hard to define precisely when a child (or an adult) has put on too many pounds. But, chances are, there's no hiding those superfluous pounds, especially from yourself. If your child is overweight, trust me, he or she will know it without having to be told.

Being overweight for a child can be a chilling experience. The quality of mercy can be practically nonexistent in children. The level of taunting that goes on can be frightening. Tragically enough, several years ago things got to the point of desperation for one poor child. He couldn't bear going to school any longer where he was being called names by his classmates. Obviously in deep pain, he was driven to commit suicide. This particular child lacked the necessary support systems either at home or at school to prevent this tragedy. Unfortunately, this was not an isolated and extreme incident. This is becoming a worldwide phenomenon, with a girl suffering this same fate recently in England.

"who am I?"

Proper self-image is critical to a child's development. Think about it. If you were a good athlete as a child, you will probably always think of yourself as being so. And if you did well academically, you will probably always think of yourself as being smart. By the same token, if you were fat as a child, no matter how thin you may be as an adult, you can be sure that the perception you have of yourself is always going to be that you're fat. I still suffer from the thought that I am overweight, despite the fact that I carry only 165 pounds on my six-foot frame. I look into the mirror and I see the overweight child staring back at me. And no matter how thin I am, it is something that will probably never change.

Recent studies have shown that children who lose weight gain an enormous amount of self-esteem. If you ask many of the overweight adult patients that I treat, you'll inevitably find that one of their main motivating factors is the self-esteem they will gain. Of course, they don't actually say it in those words. Instead, they'll usually say, "I want to look better in my clothes," or "I want my wife to find me attractive again."

It's the same for children, only they use different words to express the same hopes. I hear phrases like, "I want to be just like my best friend," or, "I want to hang out at the mall like Mike." It's a little more difficult to "hear" what they're saying, yet the emotion remains the same: they want to lose weight so they can feel better about themselves.

boys and girls

The differences between boys and girls in the area of self-esteem is noteworthy. In a survey conducted by the Commonwealth Fund, in which 3,586 girls and 3,162 boys from grades five through twelve were interviewed, it was found that there was a marked difference in the self-perception between the sexes.

This survey found that young girls entering puberty experience a crisis in confidence that renders them vulnerable to risky health behaviors, such as alcohol consumption, drug use, and eating disorders. Dr. Emily Hancock, a psychologist and author of *The Girl Within*, shows that self-esteem in girls peaks at the age of nine, then begins to plummet. Backing up this contention, the Fund study reports that by high school, only 39 percent of girls were highly self-confident and that older girls had less self-confidence than younger girls.

Another interesting finding from this survey is that older boys were more likely to be highly self-confident than younger boys, with more than half of all boys in high school indicating high self-confidence. I'd bet that it was the boys who were overweight who displayed lower self-confidence.

Something else from this study that caught my eye was that girls were particularly likely to be critical of themselves and 25 percent of older girls reported that they did not like themselves, whereas only 14 percent of the boys felt this way.

The Fund survey reported that many nine-year-olds are dieting to lose weight. Furthermore, up to 25 percent of adolescents, many of them girls, regularly purge themselves to control their weight. In fact, nearly one in five ninth-grade girls admitted to having binged and purged, and the incidence of bulimia is twice that amongst high school seniors.

I see these statistics as a cry for help. Our children don't know where to turn for guidance. One place they often turn to, the media, frequently gives them damaging advice. When there is a television special on models—many of whom are teens themselves—one of the most often asked questions to them is "What do you eat?" or "How do you stay so thin?" Children will hear what the models say and use it as gospel. Let's face it, do we really want our children to get nutritional advice from another adolescent? There are also many programs that deal with eating disorders. When these shows air, many girls report seeing the troubled girls on television as having desirable weights, and they long to be like them. The only way they know how, however, is to develop an eating disorder themselves.

By losing weight and gaining health, there is no end to the amount of self-esteem that can be gained. Giving children something they can do for themselves in terms of nutrition that they know is right gives them self-esteem just by knowing they've made the right decisions when it comes to food. That in and of itself can help to raise self-esteem levels to new heights. Just think of what all that self-confidence can bring. Now your kids can have it all and be healthy at the same time.

can I keep my child on a diet?

One day I received a call from the mother of one of my young patients named Jason. Jason was about to go to his first birthday party as a dieter, and his mother was concerned not only about how Jason would deal with his diet in those surroundings, but also about how his peers would react to his special diet. After thinking about it for a while, I decided that the best solution would be to have Jason's mom call the other child's mother and explain to her that Jason was on a special diet and that she would like to send over something special for him to snack on. Of course, it was fine with the birthday boy's mother. I gave Jason's mom a list of fun foods he could bring with him so he wouldn't feel as if he were being left out. In the end, the food I had her prepare was so delicious that all the other kids wanted to eat just what Jason had. Certainly, I can't guarantee that all life's difficult situations can be resolved this easily, but I do know that dieting is always more successful when there is some thought involved.

One of the great fears expressed by parents is that they doubt that *their* child can stay on a diet. "Dr. Pescatore," they say, "I can't be with them all the time. How can I make sure that they eat what's good for them?"

The truth is, children don't want to be overweight. They want to lose weight so they will feel better, look better, and, most importantly, fit in with their peers. Too many parents underestimate their children. In my experience, children are often more motivated and more disciplined than their parents. A child, for the most part, will do what he or she is told. They generally accept authority, and they are looking for structure that only you, as a parent, can provide. They generally accept the dietary limitations placed on them. I can't say the same for my adult patients, who offer excuse after excuse as to why they can't stay on their diet.

From my experience, as soon as children begin losing weight on the diet, a natural reinforcement begins to take place. They begin to feel better about themselves. They begin to relate better to their peers. And, in my experience, they often choose to stay on the weight-loss part of the diet far longer than they have to. A better self-image is starting to take hold, and they are very reluctant to give this up. A positive self-image can be just as self-perpetuating as a negative self-image, and often even more so.

like father like son, like mother like daughter

It happens all the time. In talking about their overweight child, a mother or father will inevitably shrug his or her shoulders and say, "What can we do about it? I'm fat. My wife's fat. Why should our children be any different?" Or I have even heard the opposite. "Dr.

Pescatore, I don't understand it. I'm thin. My husband's thin. How can our son be fat?"

The answer is simple: biology is not always destiny, even though it may often appear to turn out that way. If it were, today I would weigh far more than 165 pounds.

I say this despite the plethora of medical reports that surface from time to time saying how genetics plays a major role in determining obesity. For instance, a recent study published in the *New England Journal of Medicine* found that among children under the age of ten, having an overweight parent roughly doubled the child's risk of becoming a heavy adult, even if the youngster was normal in size. Dr. Robert Whitaker of Children's Hospital Medical Center in Cincinnati, a co-author of the study, went so far as to say, "Normal weight parents don't have to worry about their heavy toddler growing up to be an obese adult."

I disagree with the findings of this study, and I worry about the implications for the normal-weight adult with an overweight child under the age of ten. It may lead them to think they do not have anything to worry about, and as a result, they may feed their child anyway they like. It also leads the overweight family of an overweight ten-year-old to just give up.

Obesity runs in families both because children inherit a genetic tendency to be fat and because families share eating and exercise habits that may make them put on weight. This study suggests that genes probably start to exert their influence early in life, while individual behavior plays a bigger role as youngsters get older.

By the time a child is ten years old, it is the child's own weight that appears to be the major determining factor of later obesity. I believe it is never too early to begin to be concerned with your child's weight and overall health, and I don't want parents to be misled by statements that encourage the status quo.

One example I like to use with my patients is the analogy of the seed (genetics) that falls into the soil (the environment). If the soil is rich in nutrients, the seed will blossom (as will your child's waistline). If the soil does not promote the growth of the seed, then obviously it will not blossom. Consequently, we have a two-pronged sword. We don't want the seed to blossom too much, resulting in obesity, and yet we don't want it to wither and die away. Children with overweight parents may be predisposed to being overweight themselves, but if the environment is not right for this to happen, then they will not become overweight. It is only if you allow a poor nutritional environment to exist in your household that you will doom your child to a lifetime of poor eating habits.

About thirty years ago, a series of studies defined *obesity* at the cellular level. The investigators showed that fat may be packaged in the body in two ways: either in small droplets contained in many fat cells or in large drops contained in a few fat cells. In this way, they were able to distinguish between two types of obesity: *hyperplastic obesity*, in which there were too many fat cells, but each contains a relatively normal amount of fat (childhood obesity, they found, was invariably of the hyperplastic variety); and *hypertrophic obesity*, in which there is a normal amount of fat cells, but each contains too much fat.

Furthermore, they found that weight loss always reduced the amount of fat per cell, but never the number of fat cells. Consequently, the person who had hypertrophic obesity (fewer fat cells with more fat in each one) was returned to normal when he or she lost weight. In contrast, the person who had hyperplastic obesity (too many fat cells) was made doubly abnormal with weight reduction. Now, this person had too many small fat cells and, as a result, weight gain and eventual return to obesity were almost inevitable.

Over the past few years, several studies have been conducted that have shown that the *heritability* (i.e., how likely body fatness and body-fat distribution is related to a genetic component) is approximately 65 percent. So you can see that it is *not* inevitable that an obese parent will produce an obese child.

In the ten to fifteen years after these findings were first published, other studies were designed to discover whether treatment for one kind of obesity should be different from treatment for the other. The results of all these studies were essentially the same: (1) weight loss is difficult to maintain, no matter what kind of obesity you have; but (2) a proper diet, along with exercise, will cure obesity. This is great news, but the question remains: *what, exactly, is a proper diet?*

The United States Department of Agriculture, among others, has provided low-fat, high-carbohydrate dietary guidelines. As a result of these guidelines, the current dietary-fat and saturated-fat intake of American children is lower than in the past. Nonetheless, in the thirty years since the original studies on fat cells were published, the rate of childhood obesity has doubled.

"I don't like it!"

It's true that as a general rule children don't like to try new foods and will often say they hate them. Nevertheless, I can promise you, that if you put a food on the table often enough, they'll eventually eat it and even begin to like it. This conclusion comes from years of experience with parents and their children. I've had so many parents say to me, after their child has been on my diet for a period of time, that they are so surprised to see their child eat vegetables. "I didn't think he liked cauliflower," they might say. Children are a constant source of amazement, and you won't believe what they're capable of until you give them the opportunity to prove it to you.

Variety is such an important part of everyone's diet, but especially for our kids. They are learning so much about the world every day. It's up to us to broaden and enrich their lives as much as we can. That holds true for foods as well. I've already mentioned how important I feel it is to vary your child's diet. It should offer various types of foods. For example, you shouldn't serve chicken or fish every day. And you shouldn't be afraid to try some of the more exotic foods I will mention in this book, like spelt, kamut, and other strange-sounding grain products.

My patients generally try to make eating an adventure, and sometimes to that end we play "stump the doctor." They have to go into a store and try to find a food product with which I'm not familiar but that is still on their diet. The kids really enjoy this game, and so do I, because I get to learn about food items I may not have known about and can share with other patients. This also allows your child to become an active player in the diet, and, more importantly, it teaches them that there are other satisfying but infinitely more healthy foods available than the ones they may be used to.

Children are creatures of habit, just like the rest of us. The broader the dietary horizons you set for your kids, the easier it will be for them to find something they like to eat that's also good for them. I was lucky enough to grow up in New York City, where every conceivable cuisine is available. As a result, I was not afraid to try new things, and I encourage you to try this with your children.

metabolism, children, and obesity

Metabolism is the driving force of the body. It's not unlike the computer in "Star Trek" that controls everything that the crew does. Without that computer, the *Enterprise* is an empty shell; and without the metabolism, the human body might as well be an empty husk.

Metabolism is powered by the thyroid gland, which you may think of as the engine or the powerhouse of the body. The metabolism acts like a thermostat controlling whether we are warm or cold. At night, our metabolism turns down so that we are able to sleep. In the morning, our metabolism revs up so that we are able to awaken and begin the day's activities, whether it be to go to school or to work.

Each one of us has our own metabolic rate, and as we age that rate can change. It can also be affected either by exercise patterns, gender, disease, or certain medications, as well as many other parameters, many of which do not apply to children.

The resting metabolic rate of children is different from that of adults (this is the rate at which our body works without any additional activity). Children are growing and using their energy supply much differently from the way adults do. Because of this, there are several age- and maturation-related differences that you must take into consideration when planning your child's diet.

For example, infants require certain nutrients that are ideally formulated in mother's milk. Milk derived from cows is formulated differently from mother's milk. Calves are supposed to double their birth weight in a third of the time that it takes for a human infant to do the same. Consequently, cow's milk is more highly concentrated in protein and other building materials. It is also more highly concentrated in calcium and phosphorous. Human milk, on the other hand, contains much more niacin and more vitamin C (almost four times as much as cow's milk), and is quite a bit richer in fat and sugar than is cow's milk. These differences reflect the different rates of growth between a calf and a human infant. Infants have a much higher growth rate of their central nervous system during the first year of life and a relatively low rate of muscle growth. The high fat and sugar content of mother's milk and the relatively lower amount of protein suits this rate of growth perfectly.

Too few studies have examined the regulation of energy and macronutrient intake in children (macronutrients are essentially the foods we ingest, i.e., protein and carbohydrates). However, there are a few things that we do know. For example, a child's daily recommended protein intake (per kilogram of body mass) is higher than that of an adult. We also know that the muscles that children use when they are in constant motion—exercising or just plain fidgeting—rely much more on fat than on carbohydrates as an energy source. The metabolic demands of walking and running are considerably higher in children. And, during periods of dehydration, a child's core temperature rises faster, which means that there must be a stricter enforcement of hydration for children, especially when they are particularly active or at the beach. Lack of hydration can cause a child to become dizzy, pass out, or lose concentration, which may lead to behavioral problems, and can leave them susceptible to having an increased number of kidney and urinary tract infections.

Despite some of this information on the different metabolic requirements of our children, there is a growing trend in this country to place children on the same low-fat, high-carbohydrate diets that are recommended for adults. In some cities and towns, these low-fat-diet protocols are being legislated into the school lunch program. I believe this is wrongly trying to force adult lifestyle choices onto children without looking at scientific data that supports other options.

Don't feel your child will simply outgrow being overweight. Studies indicate that there are things that can be done to stop the obesity epidemic. If you assume children of overweight parents can only be overweight, in another generation, at the current obesity levels, nearly everyone will suffer from a weight problem. The Next Generation Diet will prevent this from happening and should provide your children with proper eating habits.

Sugar Blue

Eight-year-old Lucas was brought to me by his parents because of his uncontrollable rages that always seemed to occur in the late afternoons, often near the end of the school day. In addition to these periods of acting out, Lucas also found it hard to concentrate on what the teacher was saying in the afternoons. The situation often became so bad that Lucas had to be sent home early because he had become so disruptive to the other students. Once he got home, he would run around for a few minutes and then suddenly, as if he'd completely run out of steam, he'd lie down in front of the television, sometimes even taking a nap.

And it wasn't only on school days that Lucas exhibited this odd behavior pattern. During the weekend, the whole family would be out doing various activities, but inevitably at a certain point Lucas seemed

31

vall of some kind that signaled the end of the day for him. It o the point where the family had to plan their outings around ʌucas's behavior.

Lucas's parents were desperate. They had been to several doctors who could find nothing wrong with their son. After a thorough history and physical examination, I gave Lucas a glucose tolerance test, which I'll explain in a minute.

Lucas's glucose tolerance test was completely abnormal. His three-hour glucose level was 38; it should have been somewhere between 80 and 100. No wonder he was exhausted three hours after lunch.

I asked his mother what Lucas liked to take for lunch. There was nothing out of the ordinary, except, his mother said that Lucas always drank three juice boxes and always took some sort of prepacked dessert. The amount of sugar in those items alone were more than the glucose I gave Lucas for his glucose tolerance test; so I could just imagine what his blood sugar levels were doing during the day.

Since Lucas was not overweight, I placed him on Phase 2 of my diet, and in one week, he was completely back to normal. He was no longer being asked to leave school, and his parents could not have been happier. Even Lucas was able to notice the difference. When he would give in to the temptation to have some form of sugar, those old feelings of helplessness just overcame him. Lucas very rarely deviates from his diet today because it just makes him feel that much better.

glucose

A glucose tolerance test is a series of blood tests administered after the patient has ingested a certain amount of glucose, or sugar. The amount of sugar is different for each patient because the amount is determined by body weight. The test measures your blood sugar for up to 6 hours (the range being 1½ to 6 hours) after you've ingested the sugar.

There is much information that a doctor can obtain from this test, and I use it on almost all my patients. What I look for is how the blood glucose level responds to the sugar I've just given my patient. I will see one of four glucose tolerance curves, as we call them in medicalese. I've provided a set of graphs in the pages that follow so you can understand it a little better.

Your child's blood sugar can demonstrate a normal response as in Figure 1, a borderline hypoglycemic response as shown in Figure 2; the classic hypoglycemic response as illustrated in Figure 3; or the diabetic response as seen in Figure 4.

normal

Let me start with the explanation of Figure 1, the normal glucose tolerance curve. In every one of us, insulin is secreted by the pancreas in response to all foods that are ingested. When your child eats, the digestion of the food will cause his blood sugar to rise. The human body makes every effort to keep this blood sugar at a fairly constant level. After eating a sugar load, you can expect your child's blood sugar to rise by approximately 40 to 50 points. It will then slowly drop down to slightly below normal, at which point it will quickly bounce back to its normal level. For example, a normal blood sugar response curve reads

Figure 1   Normal Glucose Tolerance

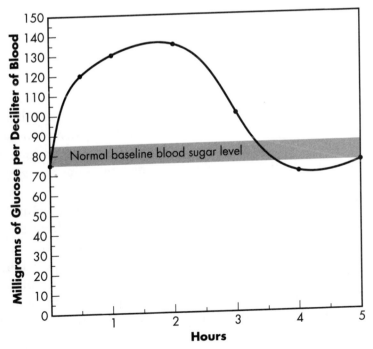

something like this: Fasting blood glucose level of 85, at ½ hour after ingesting sugar, 120; at 1 hour, 130; at 2 hours, 135; at 3 hours, 100; at 4 hours, 70; and at 5 hours, back to normal at 80. These numbers can vary, but we are essentially looking for a response in which the highest number is only about 65 points from the lowest number. Insulin levels during these times should stay from 20 to 60 units, where the fasting number is the lowest number, and the highest number is measured at 2 hours. Anything that differs from this is an abnormal glucose response and can lead to trouble at some point in your child's life.

Simply put, when you eat sugar, your blood sugar rises, and your pancreas secretes insulin in order to counteract this and to bring the blood sugar back down.

One of the many things the pancreas does is to secrete insulin. Another thing it does is to secrete glucagon, which is the opposing hormone of insulin. Glucagon signals for an increase in blood sugar, whereas insulin promotes entry of sugar into the cell tissues for storage, or for a decrease in blood sugar. In this way, the brain is constantly provided with energy. Insulin accelerates the conversion of glucose into glycogen, a storage form of carbohydrate, and into fat and, in turn, stimulates protein synthesis.

hypoglycemia

When too much insulin is secreted, blood sugar can drop below the fasting levels, and a condition known as hypoglycemia will develop (see figures 2 and 3). The brain is driven primarily by sugar, and the symptoms one can get as a result of hypoglycemia (dizziness, fatigue, lack of concentration, an out-of-it feeling) are the brain's way of crying out for more nourishment in the way of sugar.

The treatment of hypoglycemia is a dietary one. Some people will need to eat several smaller well-balanced meals throughout the day. (For this reason, your child should never skip breakfast; in fact, your child should not skip any meal.) Most others will need a special diet to correct this imbalance. The dietary recommendations are what you might expect: the removal of all refined sugars, processed foods, hydrogenated fats, caffeine, and alcohol. I'll explain more on the dietary restrictions in a later chapter.

Figure 2 Borderline Hypoglycemia

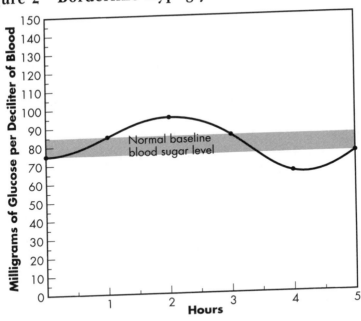

Figure 3 Classic Hypoglycemia

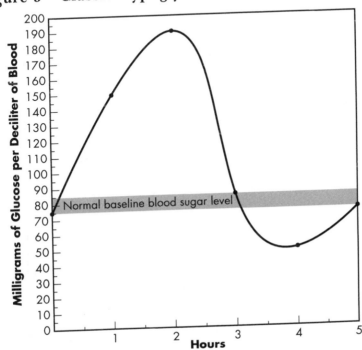

the sour on sugar

I believe sugar has caused many of the dietary and health problems we are facing today. It is a well-accepted scientific phenomenon that recently developed societies that have adopted the habits of western civilization (i.e., a diet higher in sugar and refined carbohydrates) will show a higher incidence of diabetes (see figure 4) and heart disease.

Sugar is nothing more than a simple carbohydrate. There are two types of sugars: monosaccharides, such as glucose, dextrose, fructose, and galactose (which is found, for instance, in milk), and disaccharides, which are various combinations of two monosaccharides. Sucrose, for example, is composed of glucose plus fructose.

Complex carbohydrates are formed when three or more glucose molecules combine into a polysaccharide. Complex carbohydrates take longer to digest than simple carbohydrates. Because of this delay, sugar enters the bloodstream more gradually, thus preventing a major

Figure 4   Diabetes Mellitus

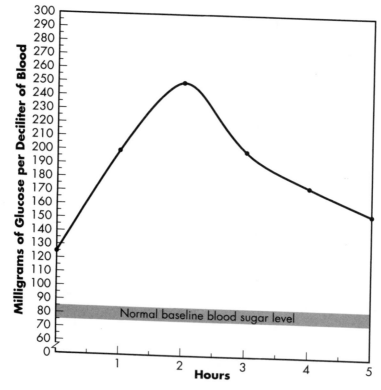

outpouring of insulin from the pancreas—our goal with this diet. Complex carbohydrates have a stabilizing effect on the blood sugar concentration and are also loaded with nutrients.

Three common sugars comprise all edible carbohydrates: glucose, galactose, and fructose. Each of these has a different molecular structure and each will be absorbed at a different rate from the bloodstream.

Glucose, by far the most common of the sugars, is found in grains, breads, cereals, pastas, starches, and vegetables. Fructose is the sugar found in fruit and in many products labeled as "no sugar added." Galactose is found in dairy products. Of the three, only glucose can be released directly into the bloodstream. Galactose and fructose must first be converted to glucose in the liver before they can enter the bloodstream. In the case of fructose, this is a slower process, particularly for the fructose that is contained in whole fruit. This is why the glycemic index (which I will explain later in this chapter) of certain fruits is on the low side, compared to foods that are primarily composed of glucose, like the pasta we are being told is "healthy." The extra step for fructose and galactose slows down their digestion, somewhat.

In most western countries, sugar consumption is well over 100 pounds per year per person, constituting roughly 15 to 20 percent of the total caloric intake of every man, woman, and child. This may not seem like much spread out over the course of an entire year, but to put it in perspective, consider that it is higher than the caloric intake provided by meat, fish, eggs, cheese, or bread. The per capita consumption of sugar in this country alone has increased 20 percent from 1970 to 1993 (149 pounds as compared to 125 pounds). What makes this particularly worrisome is that the calories derived from sugar are nutritionally barren. In most cases the sugar we ingest will satisfy our hunger, thereby displacing (or leaving no room for) foods with real nutritional value.

Teenage boys ingest even more than 149 pounds of sugar a year. Let's put this in more understandable terms. That 149 pounds equates to over 10 pounds of sugar per month, 4½ cups per week, 33 teaspoons per day. This seems hard to imagine, but realize that much of this sugar is consumed in disguised forms. For children, sugar often comes in the form of colas or other soft drinks, candy bars, preservative-packed snacks, and pastas and breads made with refined instead of whole grain flours.

When we think of sugar, we naturally think of those foods where the pleasantly familiar sweet taste gives it away: candy, ice cream, cake, cookies, and so on ("all the good stuff"). For example, 4 ounces of hard candy contains the equivalent of 20 teaspoonfuls of sugar; a slice of cherry pie, 10 teaspoons; ½ cup of sherbet, 9 teaspoons; 6 fluid ounces of ginger ale, 5 teaspoons; and a glazed donut, 6 teaspoons.

sugar by any other name— avoiding hidden sweets

We would probably agree that all these foods I've mentioned seem obvious sources of sugar, but sugar makes a major appearance in foods you wouldn't suspect. In fact, there are numerous euphemisms for sugar. For instance, sugar is honey, concentrated fruit juice, barley malt, maple syrup, rice syrup, cane sugar, fructose, and so on. Take a look at food labels, and if you see anything that ends in -ose or -ol, it's sugar, too.

What is even more striking, and perhaps even more troubling, is the change in the availability of specific sugars in the past two decades. Sucrose, or cane sugar, consumption dropped from 81 percent to 44 percent of the total market share; whereas, the consumption of corn sweetener (usually in the form of high fructose corn syrup) increased from 18 percent to 55 percent of total market share. This change has primarily occurred in the soft drink industry because high fructose corn syrup is what is used to sweeten soft drinks today. Could this be the reason that a recent study showed that children who consumed more soft drinks were more likely to be obese? U.S. Department of Agriculture data shows that teenage boys drink twice as much soda as milk and that teenage girls drink one and a half times as much. What is even more frightening is that children under five are drinking 23 percent more soft drinks than in the late 1970s. As parents, we have to be constantly aware of what our children are eating *and* drinking.

Something as seemingly innocuous as a soft drink has now been clinically associated with an increase in obesity in our children. The sugar in the soft drink is the culprit, and, in the case of obesity, it is irrelevant whether that sugar is in the form of sucrose or high fructose corn syrup.

The five top-selling sodas are also loaded with caffeine. Caffeine is an addictive substance, no less so than nicotine. In addition, it is a neurostimulant, meaning that it acts in the body like an amphetamine: it can cause jitteriness, anxiety, weight loss, and insomnia—all of which can lead to poor school performance.

Is this really something you want your child to be drinking every day? You would certainly not think twice before forbidding your child to take any other drug, so why should caffeine be acceptable? The answer is, it shouldn't be, and I discourage its use in any form for all my patients, not just children. Besides, caffeine can wreak havoc on blood sugar metabolism, and with this dietary plan we are trying to correct such imbalances.

Sugar is also contained in canned foods such as tomato sauce and baked beans; boxed foods such as rice pilaf mix, crackers, and stuffing; meats such as frankfurters, luncheon meats, fresh pork sausage links, and hams; condiments such as pickles, prepared mustard, tartar sauce, and ketchup. Some brands of ketchup contain more sugar than ice cream does.

There are also 300 standardized types of food that may contain sugar without any declaration on the label. These include salad dressings, canned vegetables, peanut butter, vanilla extract, and even iodized salt.

Yet another example of the sugar sleight of hand is the so-called healthier potato chip that is no longer fried but baked and is low in fat. Take a close look at the nutrition label, and you'll see that the second ingredient is corn syrup, and then you'll find dextrose further down the list. Yes, we've eliminated the fat, but we've added sugar to get it to taste good. If you examine the label closely, you'll see that there is now a not insignificant amount of sugar in a product, the potato, that has no naturally occurring simple sugar. Why put sugar into something that doesn't already have it?

truth or fiction in food labels

Manufacturers have found it to be cheaper to replace natural cane sugar with high fructose corn syrup. This is a by-product of the corn farming industry and a way to make more profit out of the existing crop. So what? Sugar is sugar, right? Well, for the most part that is true. However, what has happened is that a natural product like cane sugar has been replaced with a processed product like high fructose corn syrup. In my clinical practice, I have found corn to be a product to which many of my patients, both young and old, have a sensitivity. In later chapters, I will explain how I determine such a sensitivity. I feel this may be one of the many causes of the significant increase in the number of children suffering from asthma, allergies, and attention deficit hyperactivity disorder, as well as other behavioral disturbances. There has to be a cause for these disorders, and I feel it is necessary to look not only at what our children are eating, but at how it got to the table.

how can fruit be bad for my child?

You mustn't be fooled into thinking your child doesn't eat any sugar because they eat fruit. This is an important point because so many of my patients are under the impression that if they or their children eat fruit, they are eating a healthy alternative to sugar and doing the right thing. Certainly, there are some fruits that are better for you than others—any berries or melons, followed by plums, are fruit that have a lower glycemic index. The sugar is released from these fruits more slowly because of the fiber. But apples and orange juice have more sugar in them than bread, some cookies, and some candy bars.

Some may argue that there is a certain health advantage from fruit, and I agree that there is a definite benefit to the bioflavonoids—the biologically active compounds that give the fruit its color—found in the fruit. They are very healthful and very health promoting. In fact, there is much research presently being conducted that is looking into the health benefits of these bioflavonoids. However, the sugar that is found in the fruit is the same, biochemically, as the high fructose corn syrup and the cane sugar known as sucrose. When your body is trying to metabolize the sugar, it does not matter whether it came from a fruit, from fruit juice, or from ice cream.

Consider this about fruit juice. A 12-ounce glass of orange juice is derived from six large oranges. By drinking only the fruit juice, your child is getting more sugar—it is unlikely any child would sit down and eat six oranges. Therefore, your child gets all the bad qualities of the fruit, the sugar, without the benefits, the natural fiber. Also, if you're thinking these glasses of juice, or juice packs, count for the five-a-day

recommendations, think again. The nutritional value of a fruit co.
from the fiber and pulp, not the juice. This same scenario applies to
all fruits.

glycemic index vs. glycemic load

A *glycemic index* quantitatively assesses foods based on the glucose
response and the insulin demand that is produced for a given amount
of carbohydrate, assigning each food a number. The *glycemic load* indicates the glucose response or the insulin demand that is induced by the
total carbohydrate intake per meal. In Phase 2 and Phase 3 of the Next
Generation Diet, the foods your child should be eating should be the
lower numbers on the Glycemic Index list on page 42. In Phase 1, it is
unlikely your child will be eating much from this list.

The glycemic effect a food has is the effect on blood glucose and
the insulin response that the particular food elicits— in other words,
how quickly the blood sugar rises and how quickly it returns to normal. Built on this premise, a glycemic index was invented by D.J.
Jenkins, based on the digestibility of the starch. The higher the
glycemic index, the more rapid the rise in the blood sugar level. This
is important because the more rapid the rise in the blood sugar level,
the more rapid the release of insulin.

A carbohydrate is considered "good" if it has a low glycemic index. The
index basically rates foods in relation to glucose, or white bread, with glucose being 100 on a scale of 1 to 100 (+). For instance, eating white rice
with a glycemic index of 103 turns into glucose and initiates an insulin
response much more quickly than do lentils with a glycemic index of 29.
White rice is refined, whereas lentils are a whole, nutritious food. Eating
low glycemic indexed foods is a great way of controlling blood sugar.

the insulin factor

The speed at which carbohydrates enter the bloodstream through their
digestion controls the body's insulin production. The fiber your child
eats is not absorbed and has no direct effect on insulin secretion. It
will, however, act as a stabilizing factor by slowing the rate of entry of
other carbohydrates into the bloodstream. The two have an indirect
relationship, so the higher the amount of fiber, the slower the rate of

g foods with a low glycemic index, the rate of glucose
he amount of insulin secretion are tightly regulated,
ur child's brain will be fed a steady supply of glucose.
child's body to develop a sense of fullness and well-
being, thereby eliminating food cravings.

When there is too much sugar in the bloodstream, there is also too
much insulin. This acts to bring the blood sugar down, but it is also a sig-
nal to the body to store fat because insulin causes excess glucose to be converted to fat. The body has no use for any excess fat in terms of energy
consumption if it has enough simpler forms of energy, like glucose.

Interestingly enough, refined table sugar has a lower glycemic index
(lower is better) than most everyday breakfast cereals. The following
table may surprise you.

❖ Some Common Foods and Their Glycemic ❖ Index (in descending order)

pretzels	118	pasta	71
puffed rice cakes	105	millet	71
mashed potatoes	104	unmashed white potato	70
white rice	103	apples	65
table sugar	100	orange juice	65
white bread	100	dark bread	58–70
french fries	95	cookies	54–98
brown rice	94	candy bar	51–74
macaroni and cheese (prepackaged)	92	milk	49
		hot chocolate	49
carrots	92	sweet potato	48
strawberry jam	90	broccoli	45
parsnips	90	peanut butter	40
corn	88	whole wheat spaghetti	40
cola	87	yogurt	
apple pie	84	(plain, unsweetened)	35
potato chips	75	black-eyed peas	33
Dry breakfast cereals	72–127	lentils	29
(puffed rice, puffed wheat,		sausages	28
and corn flakes are the highest,		soybeans	15
and all-bran cereal is one		peanuts	13
of the lowest in this range)			

Note:

- ❖ Fruits that score greater than 80 are mangoes, papayas, bananas, and apricots.
- ❖ Fruits with the lowest score are cherries, plums, grapefruit, melons, and berries.
- ❖ Oranges have a score higher than apples, pears, grapes, and peaches.
- ❖ Vegetables with a score greater than 80 are corn, carrots, and parsnips.

Some things may surprise you by being lower on this list than you might have expected. Keep in mind that several factors other than the amount of glucose in a particular product will affect a food's rating. These factors include fiber, as I've previously mentioned, and fat content. The higher the amount of fat, the slower something is metabolized. That's why your child may be more satisfied eating a cheese omelet for breakfast than cereal. The omelet will metabolize much more slowly than the cereal. By doing this, the amount of glucose and the amount of insulin in your child's blood will be released more slowly after eating the omelet. This leads to a longer feeling of satiety, a more stable blood sugar, and a healthier and happier child.

sugar is a many-splendored thing—not!

There are many reasons why food processors may want to add sugar to foods. For one thing, it makes the food product cheaper to produce. Thanks to the generous farm subsidies, sugar is an incredibly cheap product, far less expensive than the cost of fruit. Thus, the manufacturers of jelly or marmalade reap great savings if their product is made with only 50 percent fruit and the rest is sugar as opposed to 100 percent fruit.

According to the Sugar Trade Association, here are some of the many things sugar is capable of doing: sugar contributes to bulk, texture, and body in ice cream, beverages, and baked goods; it contributes to flavor and crust color in all baked goods, as well as prolonging shelf life; it preserves against the growth of yeast and molds in jams and jellies; it lowers the freezing point in frozen desserts, thereby slowing the freezing process, which promotes a smooth, creamy consistency; it protects frozen and canned fruits from browning and withering; it softens acidity and contributes to "mouthfeel" in salad dressing, tomato sauce and ketchup.

Mouthfeel is how something feels in your mouth. It has something to do with taste, but it really has more to do with the consistency of the food. Here's an example that might help you understand what mouthfeel is. Compare Ben and Jerry's or Häagen-Dazs brand ice creams with a supermarket brand or a frozen yogurt, or even ice cream you may have made yourself. You'll see that there's a definite difference, and this is due to the consistency, or, as it's defined in the industry, mouthfeel. The two components of food that contribute the most to this are fat and sugar. Over the past several years, many products have been advertised as reduced-fat, fat-free, or low-fat. However, when food processors reduce the amount of fat, mouthfeel is reduced. To restore this mouthfeel, they usually increase the sugar content as they decrease the fat content. This extra sugar will be converted to saturated fats by the body, and an entire cascade of events takes place, none of which are particularly healthy for your child.

This table illustrates just how much sugar there is in some very common food products. Many people can't fathom how the average teenage boy can eat 33 teaspoons of sugar a day, but just a look at this table and it's easy to see how this happens.

❖ Sweet Foods Kids Commonly Enjoy ❖

Food	Amount	Sugar Content (Tsps)
BEVERAGES		
Gatorade	8 ounces	3.3
Ovaltine Malt Flavoring	4–5 teaspoons	4.3
Nestea Iced Tea, presweetened	8 ounces	5.7
Nestle's Hot Cocoa Mix	1 ounce	5.8
Kool-Aid, presweetened	8 ounces	6.0
Carnation Chocolate Slender	10 ounces	6.3
Hawaiian Punch	8 ounces	6.5
Hi-C Grape Drink	8 ounces	7.3
Tang	8 ounces	7.6
Canada Dry Ginger Ale	12 ounces	8.0
Coca-Cola	12 ounces	9.8

Pepsi-Cola	12 ounces	10.0
Mountain Dew	12 ounces	11.0
Shasta Orange Soda	12 ounces	11.8
BREAKFAST CEREALS		
Lucky Charms	1 ounce	2.8
Cocoa Puffs	1 ounce	2.8
Sugar Frosted Flakes	1 ounce	2.8
Sugar Corn Pops	1 ounce	3.0
Cap'n Crunch	1 ounce	3.0
Fruit Loops	1 ounce	3.3
Apple Jacks	1 ounce	3.5
Quaker Instant Oatmeal, Cinnamon and Spice	1.5 ounces	3.5
Quaker Instant Oatmeal, Maple and Brown Sugar	1.5 ounces	4.3
CAKES		
cupcakes with icing	2.5 inches	3.2
gingerbread, no icing	2.3 ounces	4.1
Hostess Twinkie	1	4.8
angel food cake, no icing	3.2 ounces	6.8
Sara Lee Chocolate Cake	3.2 ounces	7.9
black forest cake	3.2 ounces	10.0
CANDY		
M&Ms, peanut	14	3.0
M&Ms, plain	31	3.5
Reese's Peanut Butter Cup	1.6 ounces	4.8
marshmallows	4 large	5.3
jelly beans	10	6.6
CANDY BARS		
Hershey's Milk Chocolate w/almonds	1 ounce	3.2
Nestle's Crunch	1 ounce	3.2
Hershey's Milk Chocolate	1 ounce	3.4
Milky Way	1 ounce	3.9
DAIRY PRODUCTS		
Heinz Custard Pudding (baby food)	4.5 ounces	3.9
Dannon low-fat yogurt, flavored	1 cup	4.2

vanilla ice milk	1 cup	5.4
Dannon frozen yogurt, vanilla	1 cup	5.6
vanilla ice cream	1 cup	5.8
Dannon low-fat yogurt, w/fruit	1 cup	6.0
Dannon frozen yogurt, w/fruit	1 cup	7.4
thick shake	11 ounces	9.6
ice cream sandwich	1 cup	19.0

FRUITS AND VEGETABLES (CANNED)

cream-style corn	0.5 cup	1.5
peaches in light syrup	0.5 cup	2.3
pineapple in heavy syrup	0.5 cup	3.0
sweet potatoes in syrup	0.5 cup	3.1
pears in heavy syrup	0.5 cup	3.6
beets in sweetened sauce	0.5 cup	3.8
peaches in heavy syrup	0.5 cup	4.3

OTHER DESSERTS AND SNACKS

jelly doughnut	1.8 ounces	1.7
glazed doughnut	1.5 ounces	1.8
Heinz Dutch Apple Dessert (baby food)	4.5 ounces	2.2
eclair with icing	3.5 ounces	2.8
blueberry or cherry Pop-Tart	1.8 ounces	3.3
chocolate pudding from mix	0.5 cup	4.1
Jell-O, sweetened	0.5 cup	4.2
Hunts Snack Pack, vanilla	4.25 ounces	4.4
Popsicle	1	4.5
frosted chocolate fudge Pop-Tart	0.5 cup	4.5
sherbet	0.5 cup	6.7
caramel apple	1	7.6

PIES

pumpkin	4.6 ounces	3.6
cherry	4.6 ounces	4.4
peach	4.6 ounces	4.5
apple	4.6 ounces	4.9
lemon meringue	4.6 ounces	7.8
pecan	4.6 ounces	12.0

Reprinted from CSPI's Sugar Scoreboard, available from the Center for Science in the Public Interest, 1875 Connecticut Avenue, NW, Suite 300, Washington, DC, 20009-5728.

are artificial sweeteners
a necessary evil?

I do not favor the regular, habitual use of artificial sweeteners for children. The majority of these sweeteners are chemical, and there is no way of knowing the long-term side effects of prolonged consumption.

But because kids will be kids and they love sweets, I do recommend the occasional use of artificial sweeteners as a special treat. You will notice that at the end of this book, I have listed recipes that call for artificial sweeteners. I list these simply because many children are in the habit of having sweet things, and I would rather your child have a minimal amount of artificial sweetener than to have a lot of sugar.

Since 1970, the use of artificial sweeteners has jumped from about 5 pounds per person per year to 25 pounds in 1991. Despite this, there has been no decrease in the amount of sugar consumed per person during the same period. In fact, there has been an increase in sugar consumption during the same period, and so we can see that America's sweet tooth is growing at an alarming rate.

Over the years, we've seen a lot of artificial sweeteners come and go. I can remember cyclamates (can you?), and then there was saccharin. After widespread use, these were both accused of causing cancer in laboratory test animals, and cyclamates were even taken off the market in the United States, despite its continued use without any seeming health repercussions throughout Europe. Saccharin has been delegated as the poor relation in comparison to aspartame in its use in this country, but it is still available in the pink packets. Cyclamates and saccharin are still routinely sold in Europe and around the world, apparently without a marked increase in the incidence of cancers in those countries.

A recent report in the *Wall Street Journal* questions the dangers of saccharin, and, in fact, the National Institutes of Health recently considered removing it from its list of suspected carcinogens. By one vote, it will remain on the list. However, Dr. Samuel Cohen, a pathologist at the University of Nebraska who did the original rat studies, testified that human urine was vastly different from rat urine and does not react with saccharin in the same way. In my opinion, saccharin is a safer artificial sweetener than aspartame, and in the recipes I include in the back of this book, it is the one I use.

aspartame: NutraSweet—or sorry?

By far the most popular artificial sweetener is aspartame or NutraSweet, its trade name. It is by far the most prevalent artificial sweetener in use today in most parts of the world.

Aspartame is comprised of phenylalanine, aspartic acid, and methanol (wood alcohol). Methanol, when it is broken down by the body, turns into formaldehyde, a chemical used to preserve dead bodies. Numerous symptoms associated with the use of aspartame have been reported to the Food and Drug Administration (FDA) and the Aspartame Consumer Safety Network. These symptoms include gastrointestinal problems, headaches, rashes, depression, seizures, memory loss, blurred vision, blindness, slurred speech, and other neurological disorders.

Aspartame contains a neurotransmitter (phenylalanine), one of the chemicals manufactured and used by the brain. Because of this, it is believed by some experts to cause brain lesions by literally exciting some brain cells to death. Aspartame cannot be used by people with phenylketonuria—a disorder of metabolism whereby a person is unable to metabolize amino acids and neurotransmitters, thus leading to an overproduction of these substances.

Dr. Russell Blaylock, an aspartame critic and associate professor of neurosurgery at the Medical University of Mississippi, goes so far as to believe that aspartame can lead to the development of certain neurodegenerative diseases and brain tumors.

a safe sweet alternative

I believe there is a safe alternative to these artificial sweeteners: stevia, a plant many times sweeter than sugar that has been used safely for hundreds of years to sweeten and flavor beverages and foods without adding any calories. It is a plant native to Paraguay, but it has recently been farmed in China, Thailand, and Canada.

In Paraguay, stevia has been used as a remedy for diabetes. In Brazil, it is used in many dental preparations and dietetic products. In Brazil, before a certain soft drink manufacturer would build a processing plant, the manufacturer insisted that aspartame be the sweetener in the diet beverages. The Brazilian government would have preferred stevia be used in its stead. However, the plant would not be built unless this concession was made and now diet beverages are made with aspartame in Brazil, rather than with the naturally occurring stevia that grows in Brazil. Hence, the interests of Big Business won over the interests of health. Fortunately, this did not happen in Japan which is where we have the best example of stevia's use.

Stevia has been widely used in Japan now for the past two decades. There has not been a single report in the scientific or medical literature of an adverse reaction. Stevia is used in Japan the way we use aspartame. It is the sweetener in everything from soft drinks to table packets. It has been shown to be completely safe and all natural, yet the U.S. Food and Drug Administration will not allow its use without massive human testing. No company will ever undertake this costly process because stevia is a natural product and cannot be patented; so the financial incentive for this endeavor is nonexistent.

Stevia is only available in this country as a nutritional supplement, not as a food additive. It is becoming increasingly easy to find and use, and if it isn't available in your local health food store, you should be able to get it through mail order. Hopefully, one day Americans will be able to take full advantage of this safe, natural sweetener in their diet foods.

Unfortunately, sugar has become an integral part of most of our daily lives. But it doesn't have to be. I am always amazed at the resiliency of my patients who faithfully and proudly report on the foods they've found that they like that don't contain sugar.

Sugar can cause many adult health problems with roots that begin in childhood. I believe it may contribute to some of the more common childhood disorders as well. We should prepare our children for good health by teaching them the dangers of sugar, a pretty difficult job considering it's probably one of their favorite foods, as well as yours. In later chapters, I'll offer suggestions on how to make this task easier and fun.

The Great
Fat Myth

CARLY, A PRECOCIOUS, OVERWEIGHT NINE-YEAR-OLD, came bouncing into my office, with her parents close behind her. Before Carly even had time to remove her jacket, she said to me, "Okay, so what can I eat?"

After I sat her down, I spent a few moments reviewing her case. I saw that she had a weight problem but no other real medical issues. I decided upon the best diet for her and began to explain it to her parents. But before I got far, I noticed her mother staring at me in disbelief. Finally she blurted out, "How can I allow my child to eat fat while being on a diet?"

Much maligned over the last generation, fats are probably the most misunderstood macronutrients available today. In this country, we have been brainwashed into believing that the low-fat diet is a panacea for all dietary and many health-related problems. The wisdom propounded by so many nutrition and diet experts is that we should not eat, or eat as little as possible, fat or cholesterol if we want to live a long and healthy life. Parents are being told that this is the proper way they should be feeding their children. Naturally, as a result of this antifat campaign, people feel guilty whenever they put the least bit of fat into their mouths.

According to a 1995 survey conducted by the Food Marketing Institute, 65 percent of all consumers fretted about the amount of fat in their diet. At the same time, the average American has reduced his or her calorie intake from fat to 33 percent, down from 40 percent in 1977.

On the face of it, this might seem to be a dietary triumph. The current belief is that fat is bad. Cutting down on it, or even banishing it completely from the diet, is felt to be a good thing. However, there is one major flaw in this scenario that has not been adequately addressed or publicized: the official advice to cut back on *all fat* is not well supported by science, nor did it reduce the number of overweight Americans.

I do not advocate eating all fats, and The Next Generation Diet is not all about fat. There is no doubt that eating fewer *trans* fats and some of the right kind of saturated fats is definitely a healthier idea. However, researchers have never found much evidence that limiting the other two kinds of fats—polyunsaturated or monounsaturated, like olive oil—will make a bit of difference in how healthy a person is. In fact, quite the opposite is starting to be seen as true. In a recent study, it was shown that women who consumed more monounsaturated oils like olive oil had a decreased incidence of breast cancer. In another study, men who ate more fat had a decreased incidence of stroke. Researchers are finally starting to come to the conclusion that the diet of deprivation, a low-fat diet that is very difficult to sustain over the long term, may not be better for us after all.

In fact, there has been a study, published in the *Journal of the American Medical Association*, that showed that an extreme restriction of fat intake (less than 30 percent of daily calorie intake) offered little advantage in the reduction of cardiovascular risk factors and had potentially undesirable side effects in some patients. The Dietary Alternatives Study, as it was called, showed that after twelve months of dietary effort, a fat restriction below 30 percent was without added benefit. There was also no benefit in weight reduction or in glucose, insulin, or blood pressure levels. In fact, at the levels of fat restriction below 30 percent, the triglyceride levels were *raised,* which is a dangerous cardiovascular risk predictor in its own right. (As I will explain later, the *triglycerides* are the fat molecules in the blood that actually make the fat stick to the vessels and cause clogged arteries.)

short- (and fat-) sighted thinking

I can't say this strongly enough: the shortsighted thinking that tried to ban most fats from the diet has failed millions of Americans, and it will fail our children, given the chance. Today, however, the tables are beginning to turn. As a result of recent research, a growing number of people are embracing the concept that there are good fats and bad fats. Finally, there has been some educated thinking going on in the world of dietary research. And, as a result, people are finally getting the message that the low-fat diet has been unsuccessful for many people and may not be as healthy as once thought. If this weren't the case, why then has the percentage of overweight children managed to double over the last twenty years. And isn't it high time someone took a stand and looked at the facts in a more logical way?

The fact is that infants and children benefit from more fat in their diet rather than less. For instance, in a recent article in the *London Sunday Telegraph,* the headline read: "Low-Fat Food Stunts Children." The subtitle was equally as sinister in a way that only the British press can get away with: "Muesli mothers deliver a starvation diet." The article went on to say that parents have been putting their young children at risk by making them eat low-fat, fashionable foods. Two leading researchers from the University of Surrey, Dr. Jackie Stordy, senior lecturer, and Dr. Charlotte Wright, the consultant pediatrician who led the research, stated that children would end up with anemia, stunted growth, learning disabilities, diabetes, and heart disease. "Parents are very keen to apply healthy eating guidelines for adults to their own children, instead of giving them the energy-dense foods they need." By doing this, the article continued, the children will not grow very well and won't receive enough important micronutrients, such as zinc and iron. Dr. Wright went on to say, "A lot of parents feel guilty and ashamed when their children eat the fatty foods they need; however, if a child does not receive the right calorie intake, in the right proportions, its growth can be stunted both physically and mentally."

This story made front-page headlines and was discussed on television programs throughout England. Interestingly enough, the way I learned of the story was through one of my patients who lives in England and faxed me the article. Subsequently, it did appear in some of the alternative North American medical journals and publications, but astonishingly, this interesting and somewhat controversial and adversarial piece of journalism *never* came to the attention of the popular American press. I'm not sure if this was a case of nationalism or national interest. The American food industry has a lot of money invested in the "low-fat" belief system. To change that would have tremendous implications on a system that is so entrenched in our daily lives.

how fat became the villain

Every industry has its own special interest and lobbying groups. These lobbyists are closely tied to certain senators and members of the House who represent the district either where the particular industry does business or where it is based. When the recommendation to eat less meat was first proposed in 1977, resulting from a national committee report titled "Dietary Goals for the United States," the large meat-producing areas of the country rose up in arms and prepared to lobby long and hard to have the senators from their district remove certain wording from the report so that their industry was adequately protected.

This led to a similar action from the lobbyists for growers of our other major crops, such as corn and soybeans. They needed a way to use the by-products of the growing of these crops, and they found that turning them into oils for direct consumer consumption, as well as for additives to be used in processed foods, could increase the return on their crops. They began advertising the use of such oils as lower in fat (which they are, in comparison to olive oil). But, what they failed to tell us was that they are hydrogenated fats, which are not as heart-healthy as the fat in olive oil.

Nevertheless, this attitude toward fat resulted in a media blitz that trumpeted the health benefits of a low-fat diet across the board. Low-fat diets, supposedly a panacea for many nutritional problems, became the newest trend. But the results were not all good, and some researchers noted the problems inherent in this kind of thinking. For instance, Frank Sachs, a researcher at the Harvard School of Public Health, reported, "Recommendations about low-fat diets have only caused people to eat more sugar and more calories. For our society there's good evidence that a moderate-fat diet would be healthier than a low-fat diet." I believe this is because when the fat is removed from the food, something else must be placed there in order to maintain the natural consistency of the food. Fat holds the food together, and if this is missing, then something else must take its place. Unfortunately for us, what is being placed in foods is either sugar (whether fruit, sugar cane, or derived from corn) or an emulsifier made from sugar, corn, or some other equally unhealthy source, which is not as satisfying as fat. Fat satiates the body better than carbohydrates, and a diet with a moderate-fat intake will therefore be easier to maintain because it feels more satisfying.

Put quite simply, our bodies need fat, and that's probably why there is so strong a physiological craving for foods that contain fat. All fats provide energy, maintain cell membranes and blood vessels, transmit nerve impulses, and produce essential hormones. However, there is no question that there are some fats that are better at promoting good health than others.

the skinny on fats: the three different kinds

There are three kinds of fats: saturated, monounsaturated, and polyunsaturated. Each kind of fat is a mixture of various fatty acids, and each plays an important role in the body after it's ingested. The body is able to make saturated and monounsaturated fats, so they are known as nonessential. Polyunsaturated fats, which the body cannot manufacture, are a different story.

It is important to keep in mind that fats provide the best source of energy for the body. There is good reason why for each gram of fat there are 9 calories, whereas for each gram of carbohydrate there are only 4 calories. The body loves to use fat as an energy source. It also uses fat for many other purposes. Fat provides necessary building blocks for every cell membrane. If it weren't for fat, our bodies would disintegrate and fall apart.

Fats are also important building blocks for hormone production and prostaglandin synthesis. Prostaglandins are part of a group of substances known as eicosanoids. These eicosanoids are necessary for virtually all physiological functions, including those of the cardiovascular, immune, nervous, and reproductive systems. Here's an example: Two of the most common drugs in use today are aspirin and acetaminophen. These drugs block production of certain eicosanoids that mediate pain and inflammation. Eicosanoids are extremely important substances, and because the body cannot produce them on their own, the proper kinds of fats are absolutely necessary for their production.

Fats also act as carriers for important fat-soluble vitamins such as A, D, E, and K. There are a host of reactions that take place in the body that require fatty acids in one way or another. As a doctor, I get particularly concerned when I come across children who are eating diets that are low in fat. This results in depriving their growing bodies of these essential fatty acids.

fats and calories

In so many discussions on diet, there is always talk of grams and calories. The diet in this book will be no exception, so I will try to explain the concepts. The calories in food are provided by the protein, carbohydrate, and fat in food. Each one of us requires a certain number of calories to sustain our bodies for the day. It is analogous to the number of miles per gallon of gas that a particular car will get. The number of calories we need is our gas mileage, and the gasoline is the food.

Each gram of a food contains a certain number of calories. This number is the same for protein and carbohydrates but different for fat. Each gram of carbohydrate or protein provides the body with 4 calories. Because each gram of fat provides the body with 9 calories, it is the food world's equivalent to high-test gasoline. In other words, fat is the most efficient storage form of energy because it packs more punch per gram.

In order to help you understand this concept a little better, the fatty acids that compose all fats and oils are, quite simply, chains of carbon atoms with hydrogen atoms attached to them (like a charm bracelet). A fatty acid is said to be saturated when all available carbon bonds are occupied by hydrogen atoms. Monounsaturated fatty acids lack just two hydrogen atoms, and polyunsaturated fatty acids have more than two hydrogen atoms missing from the molecule. The most common monounsaturated oils are olive and canola oils.

saturated fats

The most common saturated fats are found in butter and animal meats. However, most of the saturated fat found in those two products is in the form of stearic acid, which acts like a monounsaturated fat, thus limiting the harmful effects of the saturated fats. Therefore, foods like red meat and butter, much maligned recently, are actually less harmful than originally thought.

I contend that not all saturated fats are bad for you. We need to differentiate the fatty acids that are safe from those that are not. Many of the polyunsaturated fats that some so-called experts have led us to believe are the safest form of fat to consume are terribly fragile, and their chemical bonds can break very easily, making them subject to rancidity, a concept I'll explain shortly. This rancidity makes them unhealthy for us to consume.

Conjugated linoleic acid is another saturated fatty acid found in meat and dairy products. Recent studies conducted on this fatty acid in laboratory animals have shown that high doses may actually prevent some cancers, prevent heart disease, boost the immune system, and diminish body fat. Conventional wisdom, however, would have us believe that all animal products should be avoided as much as possible. In doing this, we would deprive our bodies of this very vital and potentially very healthful substance.

polyunsaturated fats: omega-3 and omega-6

There are only two types of polyunsaturated fatty acids that are considered essential (cannot be produced by the body) and that we need to discuss: omega-6, known as alpha-linoleic acid, and omega-3, which is an alpha-linolenic acid.

Among the twenty or more fatty acids, scientists have found several that could promote good health. These are important to discuss because they are essential—they must be obtained from the foods your child eats. These fatty acids are important players in the fight against heart disease and crucial to the brain and retinal development in fetuses and infants; and they may prevent certain cancers.

Omega-3 fatty acids are more concentrated in the brain and therefore may be inferred to have a relationship to behavior. Omega-3 fatty acids, together with an omega-6 fatty acid, are synthesized in the body to form long-chain fatty acids such as dihomogammalinolenic acid (GLA), eicosapentaenoic acid (EPA), arachidonic acid (AA), and docosahexaenoic acid (DHA). These essential fatty acids play a dual role: they form the cell membrane and therefore affect the function of the cells; and they are precursors to eicosanoids, which are substances that act as cell-to-cell communicators, telling the body how to do what it is supposed to do. Omega-3s must be obtained from dietary sources such as flaxseed oils, cold saltwater fatty fish (including mackerel, tuna, herring, cod, sardines, salmon), walnuts, and some beans, and, to a lesser extent, canola and soybean oils.

EPA and DHA are thought to be helpful in the prevention of cardiac disease. They seem to protect the heart by making particular blood cells known as platelets less likely to clump together and form clots. Nuts contain alpha-linolenic acid, converted by the body to an omega-3, which seems to have a cholesterol lowering effect. It may even be able to raise the high-density lipoprotein (HDL), or so-called good cholesterol.

DHA, derived especially from salmon and tuna, reportedly reduces blood cholesterol without the side effect of blood clots. In some studies, it has been shown to inhibit certain cancers and heart disease, as well as to aid in brain function, a necessary component for a child whose nervous system is still forming.

The potential health benefits of essential fatty acids are not limited to inhibiting heart disease. They are also thought to be beneficial in rheumatoid arthritis, a disease characterized by pain and inflammation. However, for your child's health, polyunsaturated fats such as these have been linked to helping the body protect itself from its own immune system, thereby being of benefit in some common diseases that affect us in childhood, such as allergies, ulcerative colitis, Crohn's disease, and multiple sclerosis. These essential fatty acids have also been shown to help fight behavioral problems at school, such as attention deficit hyperactivity disorder.

the good, the bad, and the ugly fats

There are good fats and bad fats, just as there are good cholesterol and bad cholesterol. Now that you are familiar with the concepts behind fats and oils, let's review some of the most common oils you may be using for your family, and I'll explain my feelings on their usefulness in your child's diet.

The Good

OLIVE OIL: I believe this is the best oil available on the market. It is a neutral oil and contains mostly omega-9 fatty acids. I recommend this for all uses. It makes great salad dressings and is great for cooking. You should look for *cold-pressed* olive oil in dark containers. It should be stored away from light, preferably in a cool area. This will prevent the oil from denaturing.

FLAXSEED OIL: Derived from the seeds of the fibrous flax plant, it contains both fatty acids linoleic acid (LA) and linolenic acid (LNA) and is one of the richest sources of omega-3 fatty acids. Because it is high in omega-3, it can provide a balance for all the omega-6 oils that are so common in our diet. Flaxseed oil should always be kept refrigerated because it can easily turn rancid. It is an oil I like to use in salad dressings. It can also be used on cottage cheese in the morning as a great breakfast. It has a very mild taste and is available in many health food stores. This oil tends to be more stable than most; however, it should not be used for most cooking purposes because it will denature when heated.

EVENING PRIMROSE OIL: This has been used for healing for many centuries. In colonial times, it was dubbed the "king's cure-all." It is rich in GLA and other omega-6 fatty acids. GLA is a good oil to get in the diet because even though it is an omega-6, which are abundant in our diet, GLA is not. It is generally very heart healthy, and its use should be encouraged. I use it with my patients to help reduce the itchiness and redness associated with eczema and to relieve symptoms associated with premenstrual syndrome (PMS) and other menstrual irregularities as a safe alternative to oral contraceptives (but not for birth control!). I have also found evening primrose oil to work well in treating allergies and colitis. This oil is generally given as a nutritional supplement to foods and not used as a substitute for other oils in recipes.

BORAGE OIL: It is high in omega-6, and I use it in my treatment of arthritis and allergies in my younger patients. Again, this oil is used mainly in nutrition supplementation form. It is too fragile to be used for many recipes and should not be used for cooking purposes.

PALM AND COCONUT OILS: These contain 80 percent to 90 percent saturated fats. Many of you may be surprised to find these here because we've often been warned of the dangers of tropical oils. This is another myth I'd like to shatter. Two-thirds of the saturated fats found in these oils are the short- and medium-chain fatty acids, which are very healthy. One particular medium-chain fatty acid is lauric acid. We have something in common with the palm tree because lauric acid is found in large quantities in both coconut milk and mother's milk. This fatty acid also has strong antifungal and antimicrobial properties and is used for these purposes by some traditional, tropical peoples.

Tropical oils got a bad reputation because early animal studies that showed a poor health outcome used hydrogenated forms of these oils. This caused the fatty acid chains to unravel and did not allow for any essential fatty acids to get to the animal. If the pure forms of these oils are used, they are actually quite healthful.

MACADAMIA NUT OIL: This is a great oil that is completely monounsaturated and tastes good, too. Although the essential fatty acids are present in extremely small amounts, they are present in a perfect one-to-one ratio, making this an excellent oil for all your cooking needs. It may be difficult to find in some parts of the country, but it might be available in your local food specialty shop.

The Bad

PEANUT OIL: This oil is relatively stable, hence does not lead to rancidity, and therefore can be used occasionally. However, because of its high percentage of omega-6 fatty acids, peanut oil should be used sparingly. It is not that omega-6 fatty acids are bad for us, it's just that we generally get too much of them in our diet. We should try to achieve a balance of omega-3 and omega-6 fatty acids in a one-to-one ratio. To do this, we should limit oils that contain specifically omega-6 fatty acids. Despite this caveat, this is an all-purpose oil and can be used for cooking.

SESAME OIL: This oil, which is similar to peanut oil in its makeup because of its high omega-6 content, is all right for occasional use. It adds great flavor to salad dressings and marinades in small amounts.

SAFFLOWER OIL, CORN OIL, SOYBEAN OIL, AND COTTONSEED OIL: All of these have the same properties, containing over 50 percent omega-6 fatty acids with only a minimal amount of omega-3. Safflower oil contains over 80 percent omega-6, and researchers are only now beginning to be aware of the dangers of excess omega-6 fatty acids in the diet. I believe the use of these oils should be severely restricted and should never be consumed after they have been heated because this hastens their oxidation and hence their conversion to a more rancid oil. Most commercially produced foods and food products use oils high in omega-6 fatty acids. Therefore, if their use is limited to outside the home, it will help us achieve a closer balance of omega-3s and omega-6s in our diet.

The Ugly

CANOLA OIL: It was developed from the rape seed in Canada, hence its name. This oil has garnered a lot of press and is being touted as the new wonder oil because of its high amount of oleic acid. However, we need to look a little more closely because the omega-3 fatty acids of processed canola oil contain trans fatty acids similar to those in margarine and possibly even more dangerous to your health. This oil may be acceptable for cold uses, such as salad dressing or marinades. Once heated, because of its high sulfur content, it turns rancid very quickly. I believe it is unsuitable for human consumption in the heated state, so don't cook with it or eat anything that's been cooked with it.

MARGARINE: This is the only other fat that bears mentioning in this category. About 25 percent of the unsaturated fat in margarine is turned into a saturated, hydrogenated fat. Another 25 percent is turned into a trans fatty acid through this same process. Trans fatty acids have been shown to raise the bad cholesterol (LDL—low-density lipoprotein) and lower the good cholesterol (HDL). This makes one more susceptible to heart disease. Consequently, I do not recommend using margarine for any purpose.

trans fatty acids

The type of fat that is perhaps the least healthy for us is trans fatty acids. These are formed during the process of hydrogenation, which I will explain later. Trans fatty acids are found most predominantly in highly processed foods such as fast foods and baked foods. In a recent study published in *Cancer Epidemiology, Biomarkers and Prevention*, it was found that women who had a large amount of trans fatty acids in their body were 30 percent more likely to have breast cancer than women who had small amounts of trans fatty acids.

Trans fatty acids are now believed to be the primary cancer-causing agent in fats. They are composed of an altered chemical molecule that occurs during heating or manipulation of a food that contains fat, usually during the processing. They are one of the main reasons why processed and fast foods are so unhealthy. Trans fatty acids are commonly found in margarine; solid vegetable shortening; commercially baked goods like cookies, and chips, and most prepared foods. When you read nutrition labels, look for anything that says "partially hydrogenated," and you will have found a trans fatty acid. Because the amount of trans fatty acids are not required by law to be shown on nutrition labels, you have no way of knowing which is better for your child, the doughnut, which may contain 6 grams of trans fat, or fried fish, which may contain 20 grams of trans fat. Current consideration is being given to forcing manufacturers to list trans-fatty-acid content of foods on nutrition labels.

what causes rancidity?

Each fatty acid is associated with a different degree of rancidity, depending upon the conditions. Rancidity is what occurs to fats during high-temperature refining and the process of hydrogenation. Hydrogenation is what makes them have a longer shelf life, but it does not enable *you* to have a longer shelf life and may, in fact, actually lead to a decrease in life expectancy for people who consume too much of these rancid oils.

Rancid oils are characterized by free radicals in their composition. If you read any health publications, you are probably aware of how detrimental free-radical formation is in the body. Free radicals contribute to cellular destruction and can cause damage to the DNA strands in the cells (the genetic component), leading to premature aging and tumors, as well as to autoimmune and other destructive diseases. Free-radical formation has been associated with many body-damaging processes (e.g., this is what causes sun damage when we've been in the sun too long), and we should make an attempt to avoid the formation of these in our bodies.

I actively promote the taking of antioxidants such as vitamin C and vitamin E, two potent antioxidants that will help stop or slow the process of free-radical formation in the body.

processing hurts

The real harm from dietary fats comes as a result of the processing they go through. Food-processing methods, such as hydrogenation, change polyunsaturated fats into more-saturated fats. This is done to promote shelf stability, but this processing also creates detrimental trans fatty acids (it has been well-documented that these trans fatty acids not only increase a woman's risk of breast cancer, but can increase the risk of coronary heart disease; it has been estimated that up to 30,000 deaths per year are attributable to these trans fatty acids). It is believed that the processing of fats, not the fats themselves, cause blood cholesterol to rise. Most fats are relatively safe for human consumption until they are chemically altered so that they can sit on the supermarket shelves longer. The created trans fatty acids that we ingest then crowd out the good essential fatty acids in the cells.

There are several processes inflicted upon oils that make them especially damaging. They are hydrogenation, extraction, and homogenization.

Hydrogenation is the process that turns polyunsaturated oils into solids at room temperature. This is the process that gives us margarine and shortening. Manufacturers use the cheapest oils—corn, soy, or cottonseed (and remember, these are the waste products of these crops)—

and mix them with nickel oxide (tiny metal particles). Next, soap-like emulsifiers and starch are squeezed into the mixture to give it a better consistency. It is then steam-cleaned to remove its horrible odor, and then it is bleached to remove its natural gray appearance. Whenever I get into this discussion with my patients, the older ones in the room inevitably will remember getting this product in its original gray form during World War II and getting a packet of chemicals to mix through it to get it to look and taste appealing. Ask your mother or grand-mother, and I'll bet they will tell you this very story. Now, it's all done for us right at the factory, and we're being told that this is a healthy prod-uct. Coal tar dyes and strong flavors are then added to make it more closely resemble butter. In each of these stages, this food product is sub-jected to more oxidation. When it gets further oxidized, more free rad-icals are formed—something we do not want to happen. Sounds appetizing, doesn't it? I am firmly convinced that the appeal of mar-garine must be one of advertising's greatest achievements.

Extraction is the process of removing oil from the seeds. In modern manufacturing, oil is removed at extremely high temperatures by squeezing the seeds under extremely high pressures. Both heat and pressure allow the oil to be exposed to harmful oxidative processes such as heat, light, and oxygen (again, the greater the oxidation, the greater the amount of free radicals that are formed, and the greater the health risk). In order to extract the final 10 percent of the oil, these seeds are exposed to a number of solvents, such as gasoline, hexane, benzene, and ethyl ether, to name a few chemicals that are used and that have known cancer causing properties. BHT or BHA (chemical compounds) are then added as preservatives because nature's preservative, vitamin E, has been removed during the processing. BHT and BHA, by the way, have been suspected of causing cancer and brain damage.

By comparison, for instance, extra virgin olive oil is produced by crushing olives between stone or steel rollers. This process is gentle, thereby preserving the integrity of the fatty acids and the numerous nat-ural preservatives already present in the oil. (Always look for extra vir-gin olive oil to be packaged in an opaque container, which ensures longer freshness.)

Homogenization is what all the milk in this country goes through. It is the process whereby the fat particles of the cream are strained under great pressure through tiny pores. This allows the fat to stay in suspension so the cream does not rise to the top as it did in our parents' day. This makes the fat and cholesterol present in the milk more susceptible to oxidation, leading to an excess amount of free-radical formation. So again, a natural product is made unnatural and in the process is made less healthy.

It's time we examine the myths that we seem to hold as gospel truths, the biggest myth being that low-fat, high-carbohydrate diets are the cornerstone of good health. The second myth we must destroy is that processed food is good for us or, at the very least, not a threat to our health and well-being. The processed foods our children consume are wreaking havoc on their health. These foods are loaded with sugar as a cheap filler. I consider myself lucky enough to have been born at a time when food was still a nourishing way to obtain nutrients. I used to laugh at my parents when they bemoaned the fact that food didn't seem to taste as good as when they were kids. Not only do I now feel the same way, but I am envious that they grew up in a time when fresh food was expected and, in fact, was the only kind of food there was to eat.

The subject of fats is complex and often difficult to understand. There is so much for science to still uncover about the heath benefits of these essential components of our diet. It makes no sense to me to attempt to severely limit an entire part of the food chain (as is attempted with the low-fat craze) without more scientific discussion.

I believe the Next Generation Diet takes into account all sides of the fat story and will give your children the balanced diet they deserve.

Carbohydrates— Separating Fact from Hype

JOEY, THE YOUNGER BROTHER OF A PATIENT OF MINE, was brought into my office because of asthma and constant earaches. His mother was tired of placing her eight-year-old son on steroid medications and antibiotics for four months out of the year. She knew what I had done for her older daughter, who had an allergy problem, and now she wanted help for her son.

Joey thought he was so smart when he came into my office. His sister was already on the diet, and he thought he was ahead of the game. He brought me his food diary and said, "See, I don't eat any sugar. I gave it up when Jessica did. Look for yourself—you'll see." His mother threw me a knowing glance, and as I reviewed his diary, I saw he was right—he no longer ate white sugar products such as cake, candy, and cookies. He was a step ahead of most of my other patients at the beginning of treatment. But his food diary was filled with cereal and milk for breakfast, sandwiches on white bread for lunch, and pasta for dinner. I explained to him in full detail that many of the processed foods he was eating were nothing but sugar because the body metabolizes simple carbohydrates in almost the exact same way as sugar.

In various studies over the years, the vast increase in the consumption of sugar has been associated with disorders such as obesity, dental problems, dyspepsia, gout, and diabetes. Heart disease has also been related to an increase in sugar consumption.

All these studies present a frightening picture, and yet what is even more frightening is that these studies go largely unheeded by both the popular press and the medical establishment. Far too many Americans have opted for the low-fat, high-carbohydrate diet as safe, healthy, and nutritious. What they have failed to realize is that these diets are also high in sugar.

I am afraid our children are being turned into sugar addicts without most of us being aware. I'm sure most parents would agree with the notion that sugar is not something you should be feeding your child all the time. That's why most parents limit the amount of cupcakes or ice cream their children can have. However, these same parents would not think twice about giving their children white bread for sandwiches, fruit as often as they want, fruit juice as the child's main beverage, or pretzels as a snack, simply because they are fat-free.

read your food labels

Because most of us are now in the habit of reading food labels, we are being led to believe that sugar has been reduced in many of the products we eat every day. In fact, what has happened is the clever substitution of three or four different types of sugar so the word *sugar* would not appear as the most prevalent ingredient on the label. A typical food label may now look like this: oats, corn syrup, malted barley, brown sugar, sugar, and honey. The information that has gotten to consumers is that the farther down the ingredients list something is on the label, the less significant that ingredient is. Therefore the manufacturers try to get us to believe that because sugar is low on the list, there's not that much of it. But in case you haven't noticed, five of these six ingredients are sugar, but in a different form. An uneducated consumer would look at this label and be misled into believing that sugar is not a significant ingredient in that particular food item, yet it may be as much as five out of six of the ingredients.

Unfortunately, we are also being led to believe that "sugar-free" and, my personal favorite, "no sugar added" are just what they seem. However, if you look closely at the labels, you may see sugar in many other disguises. It is possible to do this because high fructose corn syrups (HFCS) and other additives of its kind are not classified as sugar by the Food and Drug Administration or the U.S. Department of Agriculture (USDA), and products containing them may, therefore, be sold as a "no sugar added" product.

As far as the human body is concerned, simple carbohydrates such as pasta might as well be white sugar. A recent study by the Harvard School of Public Health showed that women whose diets were high in carbohydrates from white bread, potatoes, white rice, and pasta had two and a half times the risk for developing type-2 diabetes than those women whose diets were higher in fiber-rich foods such as the complex carbohydrates like vegetables and whole grain products.

Walter Willett, a professor of epidemiology at the Harvard School of Public Health and co-author of the study, would like to see the USDA's version of the food pyramid altered such that the type of carbohydrate in the diet would be given importance. He agrees with my philosophy when he says: "They should move white bread and potatoes into the sweets category because metabolically they're basically the same."

Diabetes is just one of the many health risks your child faces if you feed him or her a diet high in simple carbohydrates. Some of the other health risks associated with diets high in simple carbohydrates are an increased risk for cardiovascular disease, cancer, and certain bowel conditions. Some of the protective qualities of complex carbohydrates include a lowering of the risk of heart disease and a decrease in the incidence of uterine and colon cancer. In later chapters, I'll explain some of these health connections in more detail.

some facts about carbohydrates

When wheat is refined into flour, the whole grain is split into three parts—bran, germ, and endosperm—and everything but the endosperm is removed. We end up with a nutritionally stripped product. Please refer to Figure 5 on page 69 to see for yourself exactly what I mean. The actual numbers may shock you.

There are three kinds of carbohydrates—sugar, starch, and fiber. Sugar and starch comprise the simple carbohydrates and are easily digested by the body. Fiber, which includes bran and pectin, passes through the body basically intact. This fiber also has the added bonus of being able to slow down the metabolism of other simple carbohydrates when eaten together.

When choosing a bread or grain product, always look for words in the ingredient list like *whole wheat, whole oat,* or *whole rye.* Even multigrain breads can be filled with simple carbohydrates, so don't be fooled. To be sure, you must look for the key word *whole* before the grain.

the good grains— complex and delicious

I believe many children have a wheat sensitivity, despite wheat being the single most common constituent in the American diet. In order to alleviate this sensitivity, I suggest using alternative grains where allowed on the diet.

* *Amaranth,* an ancient South American grain, is included in this list. This is both gluten free and wheat free with a somewhat nutty flavor. It is high in protein, calcium, magnesium, and potassium.

* *Buckwheat* is another favorite. Despite its name, it is related to rhubarb, not wheat. It contains no wheat or gluten and is high in protein and rutin.

* *Kamut* is an ancient Egyptian version of wheat that is more nutritionally complete and does not cause a reaction in wheat-sensitive children. This grain is high in gluten.

* *Kasha* is a cereal made from buckwheat groats, which has a nutty taste. It is essentially gluten free and wheat free.

* *Milo,* or *sorghum,* is a member of the grass family, native to Africa. It is also gluten free and wheat free. *Millet,* although not from Africa, shares many of the same characteristics as milo.

Figure 5 This graph shows how much of each of fifteen nutrients is left after whole wheat flour is milled into enriched white flour.

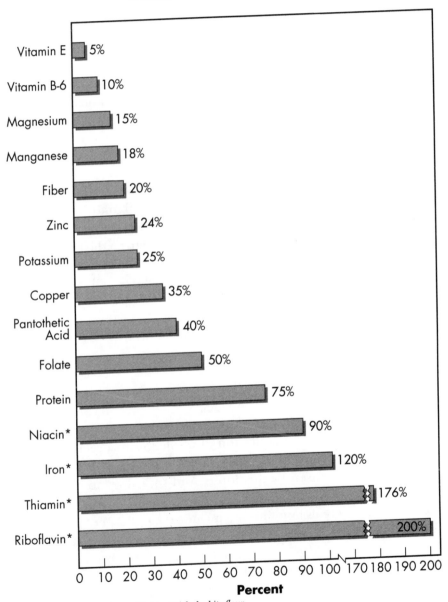

Whole vs. Refined Flour

* This nutrient has been added to enriched white flour.

Source: USDA Nutrient Database for Standard Reference, Release 11

69

❖ *Quinoa,* is fast becoming a favorite with my patients. It is an ancient South American grain and is one of the best plant sources of protein. It is gluten free and wheat free.

❖ *Spelt* is another ancient grain, similar to wheat but very well tolerated and easier to digest. It does contain gluten, but it is wheat free.

❖ *Teff* is another grain from Africa, used there as a staple, fast becoming popular in North America. It is high in B vitamins, protein, iron, and calcium. It is gluten free and wheat free.

pastas

Most pastas are made from refined flours, hence any nutritional value they may have once held has been destroyed. Thankfully, there are exceptions to this rule. For example, DeBoles, DeCecco, and Eden make organically grown whole wheat pasta made from the whole grain. The higher the fiber content, the slower it is metabolized, an all important characteristic. DeBoles adds Jerusalem artichoke to lighten the texture of their pasta.

Pasta is also now being made from rice, spelt, or kamut, which are very well tolerated by most gluten-sensitive children.

whole grain cereals

A truly confusing issue these days, which inevitably comes up on a trip to the supermarket, is the question of whole grain cereals. The parents of my young patients are always wondering what these are, and they're always confused by this topic. And so, I'll try to give a brief explanation.

Whole grain cereals by definition include the endosperm, germ, and the fiber-rich bran. The best cereals to look for are those that are high in fiber and are whole grain. Most all-bran cereals are just that, all bran, eliminating the endosperm and the germ. This will make the cereals higher in fiber, but less whole grain. I generally consider these all-bran cereals as acceptable, because they are so much better than most of the cereals our children are eating. Wheat germ can also be considered whole grain because, again, it is generally the good part of the grain that most people don't eat.

Please refer to the list below for the acceptable whole grain cereals. Also, when you're shopping for cereals, keep in mind that most popular brands contain sugars of some kind, whether it's flavored with fruit juice, maltodextrose, or one of the many disguises of sugar, so you must be careful of this.

❖ Which Cereals Are Whole ❖ and Which Are Refined?

Cold Cereals

WHOLE GRAIN	MOSTLY REFINED GRAIN
Cheerios	Basic 4
Any granola or muesli	Any corn flakes
Nutri-Grain	Frosted Flakes
Shredded Wheat	Just Right
Total	Kix
Wheat germ	Corn Pops
Wheaties	Product 19
	Puffed Wheat
	Rice Krispies
	Special K

Hot Cereals

WHOLE GRAIN	MOSTLY REFINED GRAIN
Oat bran	Cream of rice
Oatmeal	Cream of wheat (farina)
Quaker Multigrain	Grits
Ralston High Fiber	
Roman Meal	
Wheatena	

gluten or not to gluten

Another confusing issue for the parents of my young patients is gluten: what contains gluten and what doesn't and why is it important? Gluten is a substance to which, I have found, many children have a sensitivity. This can manifest itself in many medical conditions, such as allergies, asthma, and inability to lose weight, and I've also seen it in children with attention deficit disorder.

Gluten is the glue-like substance in flour that will hold bread together or cause sauces to thicken. Gluten is found in wheat, corn, rye, barley, and oats. Some of the nongluten grain products include those made with rice, millet, buckwheat, amaranth, and quinoa.

a revelation

Here's a story I like to share with my patients, and inevitably it shocks them. One teaspoon of sugar will lower the phagocytic activity (the activity of the white blood cell to halt invading bacteria) of the white blood cell by 50 percent. Two teaspoons of sugar will lower this by a factor of 78 percent. The equivalent of 2 teaspoons of sugar is what is found in one candy bar; and the average teenage boy eats over 33 teaspoons of sugar per day! All that sugar is compromising the immune system by very high percentages. The immune system's main defense is the activity of the white blood cells to remove invaders from our bloodstream in a process known as *phagocytosis*. Sugar significantly decreases the ability of your child's white blood cells to do their job properly.

Sugar can actually deplete the body of nutrients rather than nourishing it and can hinder the body from performing its necessary and vital functions. In addition, sugar can also lead to tooth decay.

Now that you know that sugar and simple carbohydrates are essentially nutritionally equivalent and metabolized by the body in the same way, it should be easy for you to see the connection between improper nutrition and many of the diseases that are considered leading causes of death in this country. The simple fact is that a low-fat, high-carbohydrate diet is high in sugar. This is not how we should be feeding our children.

the Next Generation Diet

Pre-Diet Instruction Manual 7

can I do this to my child?

RECENTLY, I HAD ONE OF MY ADULT PATIENTS BRING in his eleven-year-old daughter, Justina, for a regular checkup, as well as to evaluate her because of the wild mood swings she was experiencing. He reported that she was not the same little girl after school as the one he left at school in the mornings. He also reported that if she ate sugar late at night, or after dinner, she would become a Dr. Jekyll and Mr. Hyde. When I asked Justina what she liked to eat, she eagerly responded, "Candy, then chocolate, then pretzels, then chips." After being prompted by her father, she finally admitted to liking turkey and hot dogs, in that order. In fact, it took quite some coaching to get her to admit she liked anything other than sugar.

I'm sure this situation is familiar to many families, so I feel it is a good illustration of exactly what the diets of our children are doing to them. It also illustrates the disservice her well-meaning pediatrician had done to her. Reportedly, Justina was on antibiotics almost nonstop from the age of five through eight because of sore throats. At eight, she finally had her tonsils and adenoids removed and was able to stop taking antibiotics. But the following winter when she contracted another chest cold, she was once again placed on antibiotics until the spring, setting up a pattern for the next three years. She also suffered from asthma.

I performed some blood tests on Justina, including a glucose tolerance test and a cytotoxic food sensitivity test. On the cytotoxic food test, she reacted to candida, wheat, and rye. Her glucose tolerance test was abnormal, and in the fourth hour, her blood sugar dropped to 44. This is well below the 70 one would expect to find.

This is fairly typical of the pattern I see in children who have very much the same story as Justina. Because she was a thin young lady, I placed her on Phase 2 of the diet, while eliminating yeast and the other foods to which she was sensitive. I also customized a nutritional supplementation program for her. Within a few weeks she was better.

An interesting side note to Justina's story is that it was her father with whom I had the most contact. Justina's mother is also a patient of mine; however, she could not bear to discipline her child in this way—meaning limiting the kinds of food she ate—so it was less painful for her if her husband brought Justina to the office. So many emotions are involved when we are dealing with our children. It's important that, as a parent, you don't feel bad if you're experiencing some ambiguities before placing your child on this diet. It comes up in my practice all the time. Fortunately, the good results arrive so quickly and the patients are so happy that the parent quickly loses any hesitancy they may have had at the beginning of the program. Because of the positive effects this diet has had on Justina, her mother is now able to bring her to the office without any hesitation.

how to tell if your child is overweight: the amazing BMI

Most parents want to know what I think is the ideal weight for their child. For this I use the *body mass index*, or BMI. This has been shown to be more clinically relevant than actual weight and uses the minimization of health risks as the ultimate goal.

There are three steps involved in calculating your child's (or your own) BMI: (1) Multiply your child's weight in pounds by 703. (2) Square your child's height in inches. (3) Divide the total arrived at in step 1 by the total arrived at in step 2. That number is the BMI. A number less than 22 is our goal, and lower numbers are our optimal goals. Any score above 25 places your child at an increased health risk. The higher the number, the higher the risk. There are some adjustments to be made with respect to ages: A teenager should strive for 19 to 21; those between the ages of 9 and 12: 15 to 17; and those between the ages of 6 and 8: 13 to 15.

Here's an example. I weigh 165 pounds, and my height is 6 feet, or 72 inches. First, I multiply 165 by 703, which equals 115,995. Next, I take my height, which is 72 inches, and I square it, 72 x 72, which equals 5,184. I then divide 115,995 by 5,184, arriving at 22.4, which puts me at a minimal risk for adverse health outcomes.

One thing you should remember. Just because I use BMI doesn't mean that it is meant to take the place of a regular office visit with your child's pediatrician who should measure and place him or her on the height-weight percentile charts. This is still a very valuable tool. I don't emphasize this with my overweight children patients because I feel it places too much emphasis on the weight and not enough emphasis on health. For child patients who are not overweight, I do use the same height-weight percentile charts any other doctor uses, along with the BMI.

You and your child should be setting the goals you wish to reach with this program. I recommend discussing the BMI with your child and, if possible, having him or her figure out the BMI. It is just this kind of homework that I give my patients on their first office visit.

A goal weight is not something I routinely determine for my patients. It's always a mutually arrived at decision, and you should not choose a goal weight for your child without his or her input. I will often not even discuss it unless the patient or the parent raises the question.

If children see this nutritional program as something in which they play an active part, and they become engaged in the nuts and bolts of the diet, their level of compliance will be much higher and a more successful outcome can be attained.

how to use the next generation diet

When I first began to develop the Next Generation Diet so that it would encompass as many different groups of children as possible, from six-year-olds all the way through adolescents, I knew it would not be an easy task. It's far simpler for me to individualize a program when the patient is sitting in my office, as opposed to trying to instruct a group of unseen parents of children of various ages. After all, would the parents of a teenager want to wade through all the information that pertains to a six-year-old?

The simple answer is that much of the health information that I'm relaying to you in this book applies across the board to all children, whether they be fat or lean, younger or older. Most of the diet will be applicable to all children, no matter what their ages might be. However, there are certain restrictions or differences among the age groups, and I'll separate these into different chapters.

For example, if you have a nine-year-old son who needs to lose weight, you should refer to the general diet chapters, then go to the specifics set forth in the chapter dedicated to nine to twelve-year-olds in Phase 1 of the diet. Or, if you have a thirteen-year-old daughter who does not need to lose weight and doesn't have any specific health problems, you would simply go to the general diet chapters and then to the specific section for her age group in Phase 2 of the diet. In other words, all parents should read all the general diet chapters, Chapters 8, 9, and 10. For your own child's problem, here is the recommended reading:

Overweight	*Nonoverweight*
Chapters 8, 9, 10	Chapters 8, 9, 10
then	then
Age-specific, Phase 1	Age-specific, Phase 2

If your child has any health problems, such as allergies or asthma, you would do the same: read the general diet chapters and then refer to the age-specific chapters for any additional details. The next step would be to check the specific health chapters to see if your child's problem has anything in common with the cases of the children I've described. This may lead you to other diet variations, such as a yeast-free version, or to various nutritional supplements that I'll be recommending.

I know it may sound a little confusing now, but it's not. Just be assured that your child will be covered somewhere in this book, and we'll be able to make him or her healthier and, if necessary, thinner.

the basics of the diet for all age and weight levels

The diet plan I propose is a higher protein diet than is currently recommended by the U.S. Department of Agriculture. However, it is not as high in protein as the Atkins Diet, which has proven so successful for many adults with weight and health problems.

The Next Generation Diet will teach you and your child how to properly balance protein and complex carbohydrates, including vegetables and fats, to ensure a healthy weight loss if one is necessary or, if weight is not an issue, to simply put your child on the road to good health. The beauty of this diet is that all your children (as well as the entire family) will benefit from this treatment plan.

One of the main goals of this diet is to regulate blood sugar and insulin levels in order to maintain good health. In that respect, you should know that protein and fat act to stabilize blood sugar. On the other hand, carbohydrates, whether they are simple or complex, tend to destabilize blood sugar (simple carbohydrates are bigger culprits in this regard). Of utmost importance is that the amount of sugar that is allowed on this diet is kept to a bare minimum.

There are three distinct phases to the diet, and each age group will have an explanation that is suited specifically to it. Again, there are generalities that apply to each age group, and I'll cover those first.

- ❖ Phase 1 = the initial, strictly weight loss phase
- ❖ Phase 2 = the transition phase, wherein your child's body will begin to adapt to a slimmer version of itself
- ❖ Phase 3 = the lifetime, or forever, phase, which is a maintenance diet that should continue uninterrupted into adulthood

where does my child start?

There are really only two starting points for this nutritional lifestyle plan, no matter the age of your child. Your child will either start in

Phase 1, if your child needs to lose weight, or in Phase 2, if your child is of average weight. The reason I recommend starting a nonoverweight child in Phase 2, the transition phase, of the diet and then moving him or her quickly to the lifetime, Phase 3, part is so your child's metabolism will have time to adapt to a different way of eating, one with much less sugar, refined carbohydrates, and processed foods.

After dealing with the generalities of the diet, I will then discuss three age groups: six to eight-years old; nine to twelve years old; and thirteen years old and up. These are the categories I use in my office. However, they do not always hold true to the minute. I have often had to move children into different categories based on their progress. I'll teach you how to do this for your child. For example, a nonoverweight twelve-year-old may be better suited for the nine to twelve category, whereas an overweight ten-year-old may fit better into the six to eight category. You'll never know until you start!

The best advice I can give is to place your child first in the designated age group and then, if necessary, make an adjustment once the process has begun. In later chapters, I'll discuss specifics as to what you can do if things are not going as planned.

use a food diary

It's a good idea to have your child keep a food diary, which, in my experience can help him or her maintain the diet.

Before I see a patient, they have filled out several questionnaires. One of these is a food diary, which is a record of everything your child has eaten or will eat for three full days to a week, including snacks (even gum), meals, and beverages.

There's no reason why you can't do this on a regular basis at home, at least during the first few weeks of the diet. So, before your child embarks on this new nutritional lifestyle plan, and once you've completed the prediet diary, sit down with your child and go over the changes this diet will make in the old routine. Circle the trouble spots that will be different from what he or she is used to. Offer suggestions and replacements for all the circled items. This helps the child know she has control of her diet. It brings the child into the loop, so to speak, and encourages active participation in the diet. Remember, more often than not, during the day your children will be outside your reach, and they must know precisely what they can and can't have on the diet. A trick I learned from one of my patients was to make lists of all the foods the child can't have and all the foods he or she can have. Try not to focus on the "can't" list, and have a contest to see who can put more choices on the "can" list.

A food diary can also help identify exactly when there may be problems—the times when your child is more likely to be eating unhealthy snacks or eating outside the home where compliance with the diet can be less than 100 percent. All potential trouble spots, which may be different for each family, must be identified. Once they are, discuss with your children ways they can sidestep these obstacles. Allow them to offer suggestions for compliance, and go along with what they've suggested as long as it stays within the realm of the nutrition plan. By doing this, you make your child part of the solution rather than part of the problem, thereby greatly enhancing the chances of success.

Unlocking the Mysteries of the Diet

I F THERE IS AN OVERALL KEY TO MY DIET, IT COULD BE SUMMED up in one word: *balance*. This balance will allow your child's metabolism to work at optimum levels, thereby allowing his or her body to work in the most efficient, healthiest way.

The Next Generation Diet calls for a balance of protein, carbohydrates (both complex and simple), and fats. This will lead to a proper metabolic balance of all the macronutrients in the body.

In order to properly balance the micronutrients, I believe nutritional supplementation is necessary, and in a coming chapter, I'll explain how to do this.

control your portions

Quantities of food are something that an overweight child will probably struggle with the rest of his or her life. Certainly, I can speak with experience when it comes to this subject. However, I believe if the cycle of overeating is broken as a child, then it can and will only be easier to deal with as an adult. As an overweight child who has become a nonoverweight adult, I still worry about portion sizes.

When I'm cooking at home, I'm often tempted to cook more than what I should eat. I also know that if I do cook the extra amount of food, I'll eat it. And so, I have learned from experience to only put a healthy amount of food on my plate. This need to eat everything on my plate and then some is a definite carryover from my childhood. As an adult, I've had to learn how to unlearn that habit. Wouldn't it be more beneficial to your child if he or she didn't have to do that?

It's important as parents to teach your child proper dietary habits, which include portion control. Although there are food groups in this diet—proteins and cheeses, for instance—where portion sizes are not specifically limited, it's important to remember that your child does not have to eat all the food in the house. I recommend portion control for all food groups, if only to instill discipline in your child. Nevertheless, sometimes with severely overweight children, in order to make them feel as if they're not being deprived, I allow them unlimited portions of certain proteins until they've lost weight. Once they've begun to lose weight, they find they don't need to eat as much to feel full. It is only then, for the overweight child, that I begin to suggest portion sizes. I try to allow the child to instill their own sense of discipline because this is usually longer-lasting and more effective.

eat organically

I have tried to provide a guideline so all readers of this book will be able to successfully use the Next Generation Diet on their own. There are certain other things I tell my patients, simply to make their child's new nutritional lifestyle program that much healthier, and I'd now like to share some of those tips with you.

If you'll recall the discussion on fatty acids, I mentioned how important it is to have the omega-3 and omega-6 fatty acids in the beneficial ratio of one to one. Well, modern agricultural and industrial practices have reduced the amount of omega-3 fatty acids in commercially available vegetables, eggs, fish, and meat. Because of this, I strongly suggest eating organically, whenever possible. With organic food, these manipulations have not taken place.

Eggs

Here's a mind-opening example. I always tell my patients that organic eggs contain omega-3 and omega-6 fatty acids in the beneficial ratio of one to one. Commercial eggs, on the other hand, contain up to nineteen times more omega-6 than omega-3 fatty acids, making them a very unhealthy product. The entire healthy and natural balance of omega-3 and omega-6 fatty acids has been destroyed through food processing.

Modern science was right about the egg not being good for us, but they missed the point. The egg is not unhealthy because of the amount of cholesterol found in the egg yolk. Instead, it is unhealthy because of the imbalance in the fatty acid distribution, which has been brought about through man's manipulation of his environment. I feel so strongly about this egg issue that I will go so far as to say that if you buy nothing else for your family that is organic, please make it eggs.

Proteins

In this category of foods, I also believe you should try to feed your family only protein that has been derived from organic sources. I know this may be a difficult task in some suburban or rural communities. However, if consumers demand these products from their local markets, they will be provided. I know from many of the patients I see who don't live near my office in New York City, where organic meat and produce is readily available, that they have been able to convince their local market or butcher to carry organic foods. It truly makes a difference and because of this, the use of organic meats should be encouraged.

If the meat you buy is organically raised, it will not contain all the hormones and antibiotics that are force fed or injected in livestock to encourage better commercial yields. These toxins accumulate in the fat in the meat, and this is the main reason why excess fat can be considered unhealthy. There is a definite difference in the micronutrient components of the meat of an animal that is allowed to graze and roam free, rather than one being confined to a pen and force fed grain that we as humans would never eat. It is similar to the egg yolk example I gave earlier. There is a difference, and it's not just the price.

However, you should also be aware that not all organic meats are created equal. Because there has been no federal standard set as to what may be called "organic," there are wide variations in the product. Shop around and ask questions. Remember, what goes into the animal goes into us. If we don't protect the lower members of the food chain, we are indirectly putting ourselves at risk every day. Like any other business, the food industry is out to make a profit, but it mustn't be at the health expense of the consumer.

Animal Products

And it isn't just the animals themselves that should be eaten from organic sources. Their products, such as cheeses, should also be from organic sources. Because we are using the milk from the animal to make cheese, we must remember that everything eaten by that animal eventually ends up in the milk and in the cheese. We want to make sure we're eating cheeses that have been prepared from animals that have been fed a proper diet, without the use of growth hormones or antibiotics.

It's important for us, as consumers, to demand higher quality food products at affordable prices. If you believe there is nothing wrong with how things are produced now, just take a look at the statistics on the increase of degenerative diseases and cancer in this country. There has to be a reason for this, and while I don't blame the food industry for all our current health woes, we need to at the very least examine the role it may play in our health.

Fish

Fish are generally touted as all healthy and all natural. There are several things about fish that may surprise you and should be considered when deciding on your menu selections for the week. You must always remember the issue of balance when it comes to planning meals for your family. Too much of any one thing is not healthy—even fish.

Because of the overfishing of the world's oceans and the pollution of waterways, there is an increasing number of fish that are now farm raised. This certainly doesn't make them taste better and, in fact, may prove to make them nutritionally inferior. The water in which they're raised and the source of food for the fish need to be questioned and examined. If it's similar to any other for-profit way to raise animals, I find it hard to believe that the practice is entirely healthy for the consumer. Throughout Asia, shrimp are now farm raised as well. Just beware of what happens to food before it arrives at your table.

Another reason I would not recommend a steady diet of fish (i.e., every day) is that fish is the second largest source of mercury in our environment. Mercury is a heavy metal and can accumulate in our tissues for many years; it is highly toxic.

Poultry

Here, I would also recommend the organic or free range varieties of all fowl products. As with the other animal proteins, the bird is the sum total of everything that it has eaten or with which it has been injected. Most fowl are given antibiotics and force fed to encourage faster growth, while not being allowed to roam freely. Also, because they are in such close proximity to one another, their beaks tend to cause damage to each other. The beak is therefore crudely removed and can cause an increase in stress-hormone release in the bird, which is known to give the meat a bad taste. All of these manipulations change the chemical makeup of the product that eventually reaches our table. The health benefits of organically raised chicken should not be ignored.

Food for Thought

1. Diet foods—Most so-called diet products are not permitted on this diet. They are usually formulated for low-fat, high-carbohydrate diets and therefore contain an abundance of sugar in one of its

many disguises. Keep in mind that when fat is removed to make these products "diet," something else is added, and that addition is almost always sugar.

2. Processed foods—You should try to avoid processed foods at all times. Processed foods contain sugar or some other chemical preservative or chemical filler that should be avoided. I know that food processing is a way of life in this and many other countries. In many respects, it has allowed us to be able to feed more people than has ever been possible before. Unfortunately, these foods are often prepared with a partially hydrogenated vegetable oil, which has been proven to lead to an increased number of health risks.

3. Salt—I don't feel salt plays a detrimental role in our children's diet for the vast majority of kids. In fact, even for most adults, the role of sodium has been overrated in its connection to hypertension. That said, I certainly do not encourage the use of more salt than what is found naturally in the food, except in the small quantities required in the preparation of recipes, because the jury is still out about the possible health risks of sodium.

The New Pyramid Effect

METABOLISM IS A HUNGRY MONSTER THAT MUST BE FED continually in order to produce the energy to run the human body. How and what it's fed has, over the years, been a matter of serious debate.

Many still cling to what I think of as the outdated Daily Food Guide Pyramid provided by the U.S. Department of Agriculture. Figure 6 shows it for those who don't remember it.

In my private practice, using the Next Generation Diet, the same questions surfaced repeatedly about how the body metabolized what it was eating. Because the diet I advocate is higher in fat than what is generally accepted as correct, I needed to develop a teaching tool that enabled me to explain the healthy nutritional concepts that the Next Generation Diet enveloped. The Next Generation Diet Food Pyramid is essentially an explanation of how the body uses what we eat for fuel to produce energy.

Figure 6 USDA Daily Food Guide Pyramid

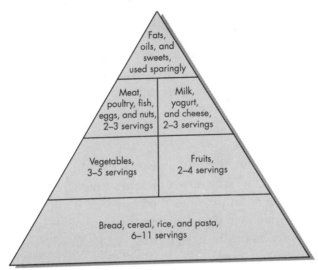

The food pyramid for the Next Generation Diet (see Figure 7) is an inverted one and is constructed in such a way as to resemble the amounts of food that people typically eat in a day.

Figure 7 The Next Generation Diet Pyramid

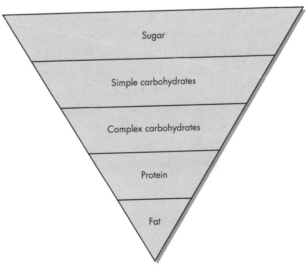

The body has preferences for what it will use for fuel. It starts at the top of this pyramid and works its way down. The substances at the top of the pyramid are less complex molecules and thus easier to digest. When the body has too much from the top of the pyramid, in this case sugar, it will use that and then store the rest to be used later. The body works its way down the pyramid, until it no longer needs fuel: If there is sugar present in the body, that is what it will use for fuel. When that is gone, it moves on to simple carbohydrates, followed by complex carbohydrates, and protein. And lastly, the body will use fat for energy.

There are several genetic reasons for this arrangement. As I explained earlier, fat is the most efficient storage form of energy for the body. Each gram of fat provides the body with 9 calories. That is more than double what each gram of carbohydrate or protein provides the body. The body therefore likes to store fat because it provides a more efficient source of energy.

When early man was hunting and foresting, he never knew where his next meal was coming from, and so he needed to store fat. This has long since ceased to be necessary. Today, the majority of us always know where our next meal is coming from—and all too often it's from the nearest fast food outlet. That fast food meal provides your child with all members of the food pyramid—sugar in the form of catsup and soda, simple carbohydrates in the form of the bun and french fries, and a small amount of protein and fat in the form of the burger. If you follow the pyramid, the sugars and simple carbohydrates will be used to provide your child with all the energy he or she needs, and the protein and the fat will be stored in places where we'd least like to see it stored.

The problem with the typical American diet is that there is an abundance of all elements of the pyramid. Simply put, most Americans consume far too much food. When sugar and simple carbohydrates are eaten in conjunction with fat and protein, fat and protein become villains. When the sugar and simple carbohydrates are eliminated, fat and protein, along with complex carbohydrates, become the essential building blocks for a growing body.

how does the next generation diet work?

Now that you know how the new food pyramid works, it's really quite simple to understand how the Next Generation Diet works. This diet eliminates all the foods that are easy for the body to metabolize and provides it with all the foods that are better sources of energy.

We are much better off eating protein and fat over sugar or simple carbohydrates for several reasons. For one thing it is more satisfying. It satiates the appetite much more efficiently than sugar or simple carbohydrates. This makes sense. Think about how hungry you are soon after eating a candy bar as a snack or a bagel for breakfast and how full bacon and eggs leaves you.

Second, and more importantly, if we eat fat and protein while shunning the simple carbohydrates and sugars, then our body will utilize these sources for energy, and we will not store them for that rainy day that may never come. This is a primitive mechanism inherited from our ancestors that we no longer need. It's not only possible but probable that your child will lose weight on a diet that allows him or her to enjoy cheeseburgers while still losing weight and gaining health.

If you eliminate the top two items from my pyramid—sugar and simple carbohydrates, even some complex carbohydrates—then the body will begin to burn what's left: protein and fat. By starting in the middle of the pyramid and eliminating the top two layers, your body becomes a more efficient producer of energy; and because it will get to the fat to burn that much sooner, it will leave that much less fat in your child's body.

The Next Generation Diet, Phase 1: *Weight Loss for Children of All Ages*

THE PURPOSE OF PHASE 1 OF THE DIET IS TO REREGULATE your child's metabolism and to break the cycle of poor eating habits. If your child is overweight, then he or she is operating as a less than efficient machine. Your child is eating too many sugars and simple carbohydrates, and his or her body is storing the fat, complex carbohydrates, and protein that they eat. Eating this way encourages the body to secrete an overabundance of insulin, a condition known as hyperinsulinism. Insulin is a storage hormone, and as a result, your child will gain weight. With this initial phase of the diet, that imbalance will be corrected, and your child's weight will fly off.

This is the most restrictive phase of the diet, but it must be so for two reasons. The first reason is that a good deal of discipline is needed to adhere to any diet. This is not necessarily a bad thing. Too often, we forget that this is an important part of leading a healthy, nutritional lifestyle. In interviewing my adult patients who have been thin their whole lives, it was discipline in choosing what they ate that played a significant role in keeping them that way. Dieting will instill the kind of discipline into your overweight child that neither of you thought was there.

The second reason is that we are trying to establish new eating patterns, which isn't easy. Keeping the same eating habits while only substituting the foods will work in the short run, but never for the long haul.

I've said that the key word to describe this diet is *balance*. There are in fact three balances. By the three balances, I mean:

1. Balance your child's blood sugar. This is the main reason the diet works and the primary mechanism by which it works.

2. Balance the foods on the plate. The amounts of protein, fat, and carbohydrates have to be balanced to achieve a state of good health. (This will be explained in more detail in the health chapters.)

3. Balance your child's psyche. This is an important lesson for your child to learn. Balance is the key to our souls and our existence. When living our lives, we often forget how important the proper balance is in our daily existence. This diet will help your child restore that proper balance and teach him or her to maintain a proper balance through a lifetime of good health.

foods to eat on phase 1

Please keep in mind that this chapter is meant to be general in nature, and so the foods allowed here are allowed for children of all age groups.

Proteins

Let's begin with proteins, the much maligned macronutrients. Protein is available from many sources, including meat, poultry, fish, and tofu.

RED MEATS

Part 1: Diet Requirements

The red meats that your child can enjoy include beef, veal, pork, lamb, rabbit, and venison. These can be eaten in unlimited quantities while still maintaining the integrity of the diet.

Part 2: Health Caveats

There are, however, certain things I tell my patients to do that makes the diet that much healthier.

❖ Limit the amount of meat to 8 ounces per day. Let me give you an example: It is possible to eat a 16-ounce steak for dinner every night and technically be on the diet. This bothers me for two reasons. The first is that 16 ounces is a large portion of food, and if your child is going to lose weight successfully and keep it off, something must be done to teach portion control. The second reason is that the fat content of some of these meats may be as high as 40 percent. I believe in a well-balanced diet, and a diet that is so high in fat would be hard to balance. I don't have many issues with fat other than the ones I mentioned in the fat chapters. I simply like to make a nutritional lifestyle plan for my patients, which involves thinking beyond the initial weight-loss phase.

❖ Trim the fat off the meat. Any toxins an animal eats will be stored in its fat, and so it is healthier not to eat that.

❖ Don't feed your child processed meats, like luncheon or breakfast meats that have sugar, nitrates, or nitrites added. Most, but not all, have been cured in sugar and have nitrates added as a preservative. Nitrates may cause cancer, and you know my reasons for limiting sugar. Therefore, deli meats are not recommended. However, they are technically permitted on the diet and will permit a weight loss. If you must, use roast beef or real turkey breast from the deli; I find they usually contain the least amount of preservatives.

❖ If you do choose to feed your child processed meats, try to find ones that contain the least amounts of the following: monosodium glutamate (MSG,) sugar, corn starch, nitrates, or any other preservatives.

FISH

Part 1: Diet Requirements

All fish are allowed on the diet. Kids especially like tuna, salmon, cod, flounder, and sole. The quantities of these fish are unlimited. All shell-fish, including but not limited to lobster, shrimp, scallops, and clams, are acceptable on the diet, and the portion size is unlimited.

Part 2: Health Caveats

Because herring, pompano, salmon, and whitefish are higher in fat, I would limit their intake to 8 ounces a day.

POULTRY

Part 1: Diet Requirements

Basically, all poultry is acceptable on the diet, and that includes but is not limited to chicken, turkey, guinea hen, and duck. The portions are unlimited.

Part 2: Health Caveats

❖ Limit the dark meat portions to 8 ounces per day. The dark meat of these birds has a higher fat content than the light meat.

❖ Remove the skin. Most of the toxins that the bird has ingested is stored in the skin, and therefore it's healthier not to eat it. If your child insists upon eating the skin, however, don't worry, it will not take your child off the diet.

EGGS

Part 1: Diet Requirements

Eggs are permitted, without restriction. Contrary to what passes for the prevailing wisdom, it is very important to eat the yolk along with the white of the egg. It is in the yolk that almost all the nutrient value of the egg is stored. For instance, the yolk is the natural reservoir of lecithin, which is one of the best known anticholesterol supplements. In my experience, I have found that eating eggs will not raise your child's cholesterol and that children who eat more eggs tend to have higher levels of the good cholesterol known as HDL and lower total cholesterol levels.

Part 2: Health Caveats

Never use egg substitutes. I believe these substitutes have absolutely no nutritional value and, in fact, may be harmful to your child's health. In order to process the egg, it undergoes a process known as oxidation and dehydration. The egg yolk is then removed and fillers are generally added to make a product that has some taste to it that the consumer would like. Whenever a product undergoes oxidation, free radicals are formed. These free radicals are harmful to your child's health. Many people take antioxidant vitamins to protect themselves from the harmful effects of these free radicals. Why deliberately give your child a processed food product without health benefits rather than the real thing?

DAIRY

Part 1: Diet Requirements

All cheeses are permitted on this diet, essentially without restriction. The cheeses that should be restricted include cottage cheese, ricotta, farmer's cheese, pot cheese, and cream cheese. Because of the sugar content in these cheeses, they should be restricted to no more than 6 ounces a day.

Part 2: Health Caveats

❖ Limit hard cheeses (cheddar, Swiss, muenster, etc.) to 6 ounces per day. Again, I give this advice due to the fat content and the difficulty in finding a proper balance. Your child may eat more and still remain on the diet.

❖ Never give your child American cheese. This is a processed food product, not really cheese at all.

❖ Never give your child cheeses described as low-fat. During the processing of these cheeses, when the fat is removed, something must be added to maintain the mouthfeel I described in Chapter 4. That something is usually one of the many forms of sugar, or it may even be an unhealthy vegetable oil. The vegetable oil, as you may recall, is usually a partially hydrogenated oil, making it high in trans fatty acids, and therefore dangerous to your child's health.

Complex Carbohydrates

Part 1: Diet Requirements

Carbohydrates are starch and sugar. Starch is a polysaccharide composed of glucose molecules. Sugar can be in any one of the many forms I've previously described. When sugars or starches are eaten in their natural and unrefined forms, they are digested somewhat slowly and forestall the oversecretion of insulin. Most of the sugars or starches in the average diet are refined, eliminating the vitamin and mineral components necessary for proper digestion and thus leading to an oversecretion of insulin. When trying to fill your child's diet with complex carbohydrates, look for whole grains that provide vitamin E, B vitamins, and minerals, not to mention the amount of fiber that is sorely lacking in the vast majority of our diets. Dietary fiber is a necessary part of bowel health. Fast foods and most snack foods contain hardly any fiber. Fiber is one of the best protectants against colon cancer.

Complex carbohydrates should be the only carbohydrates allowed on Phase I of the diet. Complex carbohydrates include the low-carbohydrate vegetables that are described below and higher carbohydrate foods such as whole grains, whole cereals, beans, and legumes. The low-carbohydrate vegetables are allowed in Phase 1, the higher carbohydrate foods saved until Phase 2. The more complex the carbohydrate is, the more fiber it will generally contain. This is good because fiber is not digested or absorbed by the body, but simply passes through without affecting blood glucose levels, which is consistent with our goal.

While there are essentially no limits to the amount of protein that may be eaten on the diet, this is not the case with complex carbohydrates. The amount of carbohydrates is dictated by your child's age. This exact point and the precise amount your child should be eating will be explained in the age-specific chapters.

Part 2: Health Caveats

There are some general rules to follow regardless of the age of your child. The allowed carbohydrates should be varied and eaten at each meal. Kids should never eat a carbohydrate-only breakfast, followed by a carbohydrate-free lunch and dinner. Granted, this might well keep your child under the specified amount of carbohydrates for the day, but it would not be metabolized in the proper way. Keep in mind that this diet is a metabolically active diet. We are trying to correct any imbalances in insulin regulation by limiting the amount of sugars (i.e., carbohydrates) eaten at any one sitting. It would defeat our purpose to have a meal laden with carbohydrates. The name of the game is balance, balance, balance.

VEGETABLES

Part 1: Diet Requirements

I'll start with what are known as the low-carbohydrate salad vegetables, which are basically less than 10 percent carbohydrates. These allowable vegetables include but are not limited to all green, leafy lettuces, such as iceberg, romaine, escarole, endive, arugula, and spinach. Other low-carbohydrate vegetables include celery, radishes, peppers, bean sprouts, and cucumbers. I generally allow these salad vegetables in unlimited quantities.

Higher carbohydrate vegetables included on the diet are broccoli, cauliflower, cabbage, eggplant, onions, scallions, leeks, water chestnuts, zucchini squash, string beans, pumpkin, spaghetti squash, Brussels sprouts, and artichoke hearts. I limit these vegetables (small pieces, loosely packed) to 2 cups per day for any age group.

Part 2: Health Caveats

Vegetables *not* included in the weight-loss phase of the diet are peas, corn, carrots, parsnips, beets, winter squashes (butternut, buttercup, or acorn,) and white potatoes. I generally allow a half-cup serving of sweet potato, three times per week in Phase 1 of the diet.

GRAINS

Part 1: Diet Requirements

During Phase 1 of the diet, I don't allow any grains except for a quarter-cup of brown rice two times per week and one serving of soy flour pancakes (see recipe section for more details) per week.

I allow brown rice and soy flour because these two products do not contain gluten, and I have found most children will not have any food sensitivities to either of these products. Also, soy flour is lower in carbohydrates, more nutritionally dense, and higher in protein than other flours. Kids love it. And besides, there may be health benefits from consuming more soy-based products.

Part 2: Health Caveat

I encourage the unlimited use of the permitted vegetables, especially the salad vegetables rather than grains, in order to achieve the carbohydrate content of the diet in Phase 1. These can provide your child with the necessary fiber that is so lacking in most children's diets, and dark green leafy vegetables are an excellent source of calcium. By freely using the permitted vegetables, your child will be receiving very healthy complex carbohydrates while avoiding the weight-loss busters. For a detailed list of these weight-loss busters, please refer to the end of this chapter.

Desserts

In the menu and recipe section of this book, you will find several dessert recipes which have proven by the test of time to be particular favorites of my young patients, and I know the rest of your family will enjoy them as well. One commercially available dessert that I do allow is sugar-free gelatin, only because kids like it so much.

Condiments

In all phases of the diet, butter, olive oil, most vinegars (not balsamic), lemon juice, most spices (unless they contain sugar), mayonnaise, and mustard (unless they contain sugar; check the label) are permitted without restriction.

Catsup is never allowed in any phase of this diet.

beverages

WATER

Part 1: Diet Requirements

Water is the best beverage for children, and it should be consumed as liberally as possible. A good habit for your child to get into is to drink fluids constantly throughout the day. I believe that a person should be drinking in ounces of water their body weight in kilograms. (One kilogram is 2.2 pounds, so to get your child's weight in kilograms, simply divide his or her weight by 2.2.) For example, if your child weighs 88 pounds, or 40 kilograms, he or she should be drinking at least 40 ounces of water a day.

Part 2: Health Caveats

I prefer a good bottled or mineral water to tap water. I believe tap water to be an unhealthy product. Most municipal water systems are outdated, containing old pipes. Potentially, there could be some contamination from the metals in the pipes. There could also be a contaminant at the source. This means that a bacteria may get into the water that was not meant to be there. This may still happen with bottled water, but it is less likely.

However, if you can't find bottled water or can't afford it, I would recommend getting an effective water filtration system for your home. This is a relatively inexpensive purchase that will last for years and could potentially save you and your family from various health risks. It is also better to use in cooking.

I also recommend flat, or still, rather than bubbly water. Most bubbly waters contain phosphorous, the mineral that gives the water its fizz. If the water contains too much phosphorous, it may upset the mineral balance and interfere with calcium absorption. As children are fast growers, it is essential to have enough calcium to help them build bones. For this same reason I would recommend still water for all my patients' mothers, who need to keep calcium in their bones to prevent osteoporosis.

Soda

Part 1: Diet Requirements

The only sodas permitted on the diet are those designated as diet sodas, and they should not contain caffeine.

Part 2: Health Caveats

I restrict these to one 12-ounce serving per day. These products contain artificial sweeteners, which I've already discussed, and many artificial colorings and preservatives. However, some children like the taste, and, I will allow it as a treat if necessary.

Coffee/Tea

Part 1: Diet Requirements

The only teas I recommend for my patients are herbal decaffeinated teas. Kids love these iced. They are permitted in unlimited quantities.

Part 2: Health Caveats

I generally discourage diet iced teas because of the sweeteners that are used and they are often loaded with caffeine. But again, if you are finding this to be too restrictive, then you can allow one 12-ounce serving per day. However, I would urge you to check the labels to make sure they're free of caffeine, sugar, fruit juice, or barley malt (another popular disguise for sugar).

I do not recommend decaffeinated coffee, either. There is always a small amount of caffeine left in the bean after the processing, so it is never truly decaffeinated. There are also tannins in the coffee and tea, which I would not recommend any child consuming.

As for caffeine, as I've mentioned before, it will wreak havoc with blood sugar and insulin regulation, and it is a drug to which your child should never become addicted.

MILK

Part 1: Diet Requirements

If you do decide that milk is a necessary part of your child's diet, I would suggest either unsweetened rice milk or unsweetened soy milk, the latter being my preference. These products are much less allergenic than cow's milk and can be used as a healthy, logical alternative. Still, I would prefer the amount of these products to be limited to no more than 4 to 8 ounces a day because, although they are unsweetened, there is still sugar in them from the processing of the soybean and the rice.

Part 2: Health Caveats

I do not recommend animal milk on this diet. The downside to milk is quite high, and I feel that any health benefits that can be gained from milk can easily be obtained elsewhere. In order to explain what I mean, I need to discuss how milk is processed.

There are inherent hazards in the processing of milk that makes it a less than desirable product. Milk undergoes the processes of pasteurization and homogenization. Pasteurization may destroy any of milk's nutritional value, and if you'll recall the discussion on homogenization from the chapter on fats, there are many problems with this process as well.

Keep in mind that what goes into the cow goes into the milk. Therefore, with grain-fed livestock, the use of recombinant bovine growth hormone, preservatives, and other chemical compounds can all further increase the potential dangers of milk.

Cow's milk is also an extremely allergenic product, probably the number one allergen for most children, and it is filled with sugar. In the United States, milk is one of the foods most commonly responsible for allergic reactions in children. About 20 percent of the population worldwide can be considered allergic when exposed to this common protein. The allergy that many children suffer from comes from the body's reaction to the milk proteins, not, as usually feared, to the lactose (the sugar). This same reaction can occur with goat and soy milk, but much less commonly.

Although milk is touted as a great source of calcium, the high amount of phosphorous in cow's milk will interfere with the calcium absorption, so your child is actually getting much less calcium than you would think from that glass of milk.

Certainly a growing child needs calcium, but there are many other sources from which it may be obtained. Dark green vegetables, such as kale, Swiss chard, and broccoli, are excellent sources of calcium. Please refer to the tables in Chapter 26 for more food suggestions as to where you can obtain calcium for your child's diet without using milk. Perhaps the best source of calcium is through nutritional supplementation by taking calcium aspartate or calcium citrate in combination with magnesium and vitamin D_3.

BEVERAGES ALLOWED ON THE DIET

❖ Water—tap, bottled, mineral, distilled, carbonated, non-carbonated, filtered

❖ Herbal teas—decaffeinated only

❖ Diet soda—limited to 12 ounces per day, preferably caffeine free.

❖ Unsweetened soy or unsweetened rice milk—limited to 4 ounces per day

BEVERAGES *NOT* ALLOWED ON THE DIET

❖ Regular soda—or any carbonated beverage that contains sugar of any kind

❖ Caffeinated beverages—such as coffee or tea

- ❖ Fruit juice—essentially fruit-flavored soda. There are very few dietary benefits to be gained from drinking fruit juice. There have actually been studies that show that excess consumption of fruit juice, a staple of many kids' lunch boxes and school lunch programs, leads to an increase in obesity.

- ❖ Milk—low-fat, skim, or regular

weight-loss busters

This is a definitive list of those food items that are not allowed during Phase 1 of the Next Generation Diet—your child's new nutritional lifestyle program.

1. Sugar (this includes honey, maple syrup, corn syrup, corn starch, and other kinds of sugar)

2. Fruit (all types)

3. Simple carbohydrates in the form of refined flours (pasta; starchy vegetables like peas, corn, carrots, and lima beans; muffins, bagels, cookies, crackers, cake, and breads)

4. Processed foods, such as luncheon meats. This includes all foods with additives—such as nitrites or MSG—and most pickled products. There are some exceptions, as I explained in the section on red meat.

5. Artificial sweeteners. If I had my way, we would not need these products. However, as I mentioned in the chapter on sugar, sometimes they are a necessary evil. Just try to limit these as much as possible in your child's diet.

The Next Generation Diet:
Ages Six to Eight

Now we're ready for specifics that apply to your child who is between the ages of six and eight. This is the time in your child's life when he or she begins to go to school and learn all sorts of new things. Your sense of total control is beginning to show the earliest signs of fading. It is therefore important to acknowledge your child's independence by allowing him or her to take an active role in dieting by explaining the principles behind it and maybe even reading some of the later chapters in this book together. This will help encourage the healthy eating patterns you are trying to provide for your child.

Your child will also be exposed to other children's eating habits, as well as the meals that are provided in school. All of these obstacles can be easily overcome if there is an active line of communication between you and your child. Don't make the mistake that many parents make by thinking your child will listen to your advice simply because you are the parent. In fact, that's usually the reason they won't listen to you, although maybe not so much at this age.

phase 1: weight loss

A child between the ages of six and eight is generally extremely active, whether overweight or not. Because of this, I allow 50 to 60 grams of carbohydrates per day. The number of grams of carbohydrate a particular food product contains is always located on the nutrition label. I would also recommend you purchase a carbohydrate counter book, of which there are many on the market, as a companion to this diet.

But no matter how many grams of carbohydrate may be in a food, it is important to keep in mind that you must choose from the foods mentioned in Chapter 10. The carbohydrates your child will be eating in this phase of the diet will be coming primarily from vegetables, brown rice, or soy milk.

the next generation diet: six to eight-year-olds

Phase 1: Weight Loss

❖ Foods and beverages allowed: Everything in Chapter 10

❖ Carbohydrates allowed: 50 to 60 grams, from the Phase 1 list of allowable carbohydrates. Remember, this is not an absolute rule. If your child does not want that many grams of carbohydrate, it is not necessary to eat that much. Instead, he or she should only eat as much as wanted, so long as it does not exceed that amount. If you recall, a gram of carbohydrate is the amount that will yield 4 calories of energy for the body.

❖ Phase 1 of the diet should last until your child is within 10 pounds of the desired weight. Depending on the starting weight of your child, this will last for a minimum of two weeks. That would bring your child's BMI (body mass index) to 14 to 15.

Phase 2: Transition

❖ With Phase 1 accomplished, we move into Phase 2. By now, your child is a slimmed-down version of his or her former self and much healthier in the bargain. You've done a great job, and you both should be proud of yourselves. Now, you're ready to move on to the next step.

I should note that there is another group of children that will be beginning at Phase 2 phase of the diet. These are:

❖ Children who have terrible eating habits

❖ Children who are not overweight and are on the diet for health reasons

❖ Children who need only lose a few pounds

Anyone starting this diet, even the nonoverweight child, will begin to lose a small amount of weight, simply by dint of removing sugar from the diet. Don't be alarmed if your nonoverweight child begins to drop a few pounds. His or her body will soon adjust to the new and improved way of eating, quickly regaining any lost weight, and continue to grow in a very healthy way.

I will now divide this group into two categories. The first is for your now slimmer child who has successfully completed Phase 1. The second is for your nonoverweight child who is learning to eliminate sugar from the diet for the very first time.

CATEGORY 1: YOUR SLIMMED-DOWN CHILD

This begins when your child's weight brings the BMI to 14 to 15. In this category, we have a successful outcome—weight loss—that we do not want to disturb. In the transition phase, weeks one and two, you should allow your child to eat an additional 10 grams of carbohydrates every other day. In weeks three and four, your child can eat this 10 extra grams of carbohydrates every day. In weeks five and six, you can increase this amount to 15 grams every other day. In weeks seven and eight, you can allow the 15 grams extra every day.

Generally, I recommend this carbohydrate level to remain at 15 extra grams per day during the transition phase. However, I do have a few words of caution. Remember that the catch phrase of this diet is *balance*. Each of your child's meals should still be balanced with the proper amounts of protein and complex carbohydrates and vegetables. Never should the allowable amount of carbohydrates be eaten all at one meal.

Here's an example. Let's say your child has successfully lost weight at 55 grams of carbohydrates a day. During the transition phase, you can raise the amount of carbohydrates to 65 grams every other day for two weeks; then 65 grams every day for two weeks; then 70 grams every other day for two weeks; then 70 grams every day for two weeks. These extra grams of carbohydrates will come from a much expanded list of foods that includes items such as beans, nuts, seeds, legumes, and grains. I will explain these in full detail in Chapter 14, as these carbohydrates are not age-specific.

At this point, it is necessary to reevaluate your child's progress. If your child is now at goal weight, you can stick to the 70 grams. If he or she has gained a couple of pounds, then you need to immediately lower the amount of carbohydrates per day and raise it more slowly. Try increasing the level of carbohydrates by only 5 grams every other day, and so on. This level of the diet will take a little care on the part of both you and your child. Don't let your child make the mistake of thinking, "Hooray! The diet is over. I can go back to eating just like I did before." This is precisely the kind of behavior we're trying to avoid. If it takes a year to build up the level of carbohydrates, then let it take a year. We are in no rush. This nutritional lifestyle will last a lifetime, and now that your child is eating this way, that will mean many healthy years.

In the above example, if all had gone well, you would stick to the 70 grams of carbohydrates each day until you reach the next phase, the maintenance or forever phase of the diet. The next phase, Phase 3, begins when your child's weight brings the BMI between 13 and 14.

CATEGORY 2: THE CHILD WHO NEEDS TO LOSE NO WEIGHT OR JUST A FEW POUNDS

This is the phase at which you would be starting the diet if your child is either nonoverweight or just a few pounds overweight.

Your child can eat everything allowed in the Phase 1 chapter. The restrictions are the same as mentioned there, as well. The amount of carbohydrate to which I would restrict your child is 70 grams per day, divided over three meals, or however many meals your child will be eating that day. These carbohydrates can consist of the complex carbohydrates described in the Phase 1 chapter, Chapter 10, as well as the ones I will describe in Chapter 14. Because these carbohydrates are for all three age groups to be covered in this book, they will be included in one chapter, so as not to be repetitious. As a quick preview, in this phase, your child's diet will consist of the higher carbohydrate vegetables, such as beans, nuts, seeds, legumes, and grains, as well as the low-carbohydrate vegetables mentioned in Chapter 10.

Children who fall into this category should remain on this transition level of their diet for one month. This diet should regulate any physical problems they were having, and it will also give their metabolism the chance to adjust to this new way of eating.

SUMMARY OF PHASE 2, CATEGORY 1: THE SUCCESSFUL DIETER

- ❖ All foods from Phase 1
- ❖ Choice from Phase 1 and Phase 2 lists of acceptable carbohydrates
- ❖ Increasing amount of carbohydrate per week in divided amounts
- ❖ All beverages from Phase 1
- ❖ Approximately eight weeks in duration
- ❖ BMI begins at 14 to 15 and ends at 13 to 14

SUMMARY OF PHASE 2, CATEGORY 2: THE HEALTH-CONSCIOUS CHILD

- ❖ All foods from Phase 1
- ❖ 70 grams of complex carbohydrates per day divided among all meals
- ❖ Choice from Phase 1 and Phase 2 lists of acceptable carbohydrates
- ❖ All beverages from Phase 1
- ❖ Approximately four weeks in duration
- ❖ BMI goal of 13 to 14

The Next Generation Diet:
Ages Nine to Twelve

THIS IS THE TIME OF LIFE WHEN CHILDREN REALLY BEGIN TO EXPLORE the environment outside the home. Extracurricular and afterschool activities are becoming more important in their lives, and as parents, you are increasingly being asked to let go. It is a fun time for your child, but not necessarily a fun time to be a parent.

In terms of nutrition, there is going to be a lot of experimenting, but it should be done with the foods we are now discussing. Make this a fun project, not a burden. Let your children do as much with this diet as they are able. Don't let it be something that happens *to* them, but rather something that happens *with* them. Nutrition is something they need to learn about, and now is a great age to do just that.

phase 1: weight loss

For your overweight child in this age group, all the foods described in Chapter 10 are allowed. Your child is allowed to have 40 to 50 grams of carbohydrates per day in divided servings among the three meals. If your child is a little heavier or less active than normal, I would recommend starting with the lower amount of carbohydrates.

PERMITTED ON PHASE 1 FOR AGES NINE TO TWELVE

❖ All foods from Phase 1, Chapter 10

❖ Carbohydrates, 40 to 50 grams, in divided amounts from those specified in Chapter 10

❖ All beverages from Phase 1

phase 2: transition

This is the starting point in the diet for the children in this age group who do not need to lose any weight or for those children who only have a few (less than five) pounds to lose. This is also the point in the diet that will act as a transition for the child who has been losing weight on Phase 1. Because this is two separate groups of children, this section will be divided into two separate categories. Category 1 is for children who have been losing weight on Phase 1 of the diet; Category 2 is for the nonoverweight or just slightly overweight child.

Don't be alarmed if even the thinnest child will lose a small amount of weight in this phase of the diet. This happens because sugar is being removed from the diet. Once your child adjusts to this, the weight will bounce back, and the road to good health should continue unimpeded.

Category 1: Your Slimmed-Down Child

This should begin when your child's weight causes the BMI (body mass index) to approach 18. We must now be prepared to tinker somewhat with our success. The child in this category will have successfully completed Phase 1 and will be a thinner, healthier version of his or her former self. This is quite an accomplishment, and I offer congratulations! However, a child should not stay on Phase 1 forever because there are two more phases they must now successfully complete.

This is the phase where you can begin to reintroduce more carbohydrates into your child's diet. There is a precise method to do this, however. You can now allow your child an additional 10 grams of carbohydrates every other day for the first two weeks. In weeks three and four, your child can eat this 10 extra grams of carbohydrates every day. In weeks five and six, you can increase this amount to 15 grams every other day. In weeks seven and eight, you can allow the 15 grams extra every day. Keep in mind that each of your child's meals should remain balanced with the proper amounts of protein and complex carbohydrates and vegetables. Never should the allowable amount of carbohydrates be eaten all at one meal.

Here's an example of what I mean. A child in this category who has successfully lost weight at 45 grams of carbohydrates a day should now, during the transition phase, raise the amount of carbohydrates to 55 grams every other day for two weeks; then 55 grams every day for two weeks; then 60 grams every other day for two weeks; then 60 grams every day for two weeks. The carbohydrates your child can now begin to enjoy are the higher carbohydrate vegetables, legumes, nuts, and grains. (In Chapter 14, I will describe these in more detail.) I keep my patients at this stage of the diet for about two months.

If your child is now at a goal weight that gives a healthy BMI, then your child is ready for Phase 3. If a weight gain occurs during this transition, decrease the amount of carbohydrates again—you should go back to the amount your child was eating immediately before your child started to gain weight again—and increase the carbohydrate level more slowly, for example, by intervals of 5 grams rather than 10.

Remember, dieting is not a race against time. This is a total lifetime nutritional program. A rushing mentality should be discouraged because that is the very state of mind that allows for all the yo-yo dieting (and the health hazards that inevitably result from such habits) that occurs all around us today.

SUMMARY OF PHASE 2, CATEGORY 1: THE SUCCESSFUL DIETER

- ❖ All foods from Phase 1
- ❖ All beverages from Phase 1
- ❖ Increasing amounts of complex carbohydrates at the schedule indicated

❖ Choice from both Phase 1 and Phase 2 lists of acceptable carbohydrates

❖ Approximately eight weeks in duration

❖ BMI starts at 18 to 19 and ends at 16 to 18

Category 2: The Child Who Needs to Lose No Weight or Just a Few Pounds

This is the place in the diet for your nonoverweight child of this age group to begin because it will help the body adjust to this new way of eating, namely the absence of all the sugar he or she is used to. It may take about four weeks for your child's body to make this transition, and I recommend that you keep your child on this phase of the diet for that adjustment period.

A child in this age group should begin the diet with a carbohydrate restriction of 60 grams per day in divided portions among the three meals.

The child in this age group may choose from any of the carbohydrates listed in Chapter 10, as well as any listed in Chapter 14, providing the limit is maintained.

SUMMARY OF PHASE 2, CATEGORY 2: THE HEALTH-CONSCIOUS CHILD

❖ All foods from Phase 1

❖ All beverages from Phase 1

❖ 60 grams of carbohydrates per day in equally divided portions

❖ Choice from both Phase 1 and Phase 2 lists of acceptable carbohydrates

❖ Approximately four weeks in duration

❖ BMI of 17 to 18

The Next Generation Diet:

Teenagers

Adolescence is a period of enormous changes for your child, both physiological and psychological. Adolescents are striving to define themselves in the world, and often that means gaining independence from parents. Children of this age will find it difficult to accept any nutritional counseling from their parents unless they play a large role in its development. From my experience, however, rest assured that overweight adolescents are often easier to work with because they often have a keen interest in how they look. They don't want to be overweight. They want to diet. They're just not sure how to do it.

Following are some of the different dietary limitations that your overweight and nonoverweight teenager will face with the Next Generation Diet.

phase 1: weight loss

This is the phase of the diet for the overweight teenager, and it includes all the same allowed foods for any child in Phase 1 of the diet. Please refer to Chapter 10 for the specific foods. Your teenager should remain on Phase 1 until reaching within 10 pounds of the goal weight or until the BMI (body mass index) lowers to 20 to 22.

A child in this age group should begin the diet with 30 to 40 grams of carbohydrates per day from the foods listed in Chapter 10 only. The heavier your child may be, the lower the amount of carbohydrate you should start with. However, I do not recommend going below this range. Any carbohydrate count lower than this will put your child into *ketosis*—a metabolic state whereby the body produces ketone bodies as a by-product of the breakdown of its own fat. Potential side effects of this state may be lightheadedness and bad breath. This may not be the healthiest way for an adolescent to lose weight (though it is an extremely successful way for an adult to lose weight). All children need carbohydrates—just not as many as they probably currently ingest.

I should mention alcohol here. Often, teenagers partake of alcohol from time to time. Alcohol is a simple carbohydrate, and it is not permitted on the diet at all. Alcohol may also be addictive, and its use should be discouraged in all teens.

PERMITTED ON PHASE 1 FOR TEENAGERS

- All foods from Phase 1, Chapter 10
- All beverages from Phase 1
- Carbohydrates limited to 30 to 40 grams per day from the Phase 1 list of acceptable carbohydrates

phase 2: transition

This is the starting place for the adolescent who does not have a weight problem, for the nonoverweight adolescent who may have a nutrition-related health problem, and for the adolescent who may only have a few pounds to lose (under five pounds).

This is also the continuation point for the adolescent who has successfully completed Phase 1 with a positive health outcome and a weight loss. Because the two groups are somewhat different, I will divide this section into two categories. Category 1 is for the adolescent who has successfully lost weight and needs a transition phase of the diet. Category 2 is for the nonoverweight adolescent who needs to get healthier.

Category 1: Your Slimmed-Down Adolescent

In this transition phase of the diet, we are trying to maintain our successful outcome, continue the weight loss a little further, and bridge the two worlds of dieting and nondieting. This is a critical phase of the dieting process for anyone, but especially so for the adolescent.

It is also the point in the diet when teens want to return to a normal way of eating. So, during this phase, we must stress the point that a normal way of eating will take on a new meaning. This means that education becomes an important part of this phase, and this will be explained in later chapters.

In the transition phase for the teenager, you may add an additional 10 grams of carbohydrates, every other day for the first two weeks. In weeks three and four, your teenager can eat this extra 10 grams of carbohydrates every day. In weeks five and six, you can increase the amount to 15 grams every other day. In weeks seven and eight, you can allow the 15 grams extra every day.

Each of your child's meals should still be balanced with the proper amounts of protein and complex carbohydrates and vegetables. Never should the allowable amount of carbohydrates be eaten all at one meal.

For example, if your child successfully lost weight with 35 grams of carbohydrates, you can raise the amount of carbohydrates to 45 grams every other day for two weeks; then 45 grams every day for two weeks; then 50 grams every other day for two weeks; then 50 grams every day for two weeks. If your child begins to gain weight during this transition, the amount of carbohydrates needs to be lowered immediately, back to the level where no weight gain occurred. Then, once your teen's weight has again stabilized, you can start to increase the amount of carbohydrates more slowly, perhaps in increments of 5 grams, up to 50 grams per day. Each child will be different, and this can take as long as necessary, until he or she achieves a BMI of 22. Don't make this a race against time and do your best to discourage this "beat-the-clock" mentality.

SUMMARY OF PHASE 2, CATEGORY 1: THE SUCCESSFUL DIETER

- ❖ All foods from Phase 1
- ❖ All beverages from Phase 1
- ❖ Increasing amounts of complex carbohydrates as per the recommended schedule
- ❖ Choice from the Phase 1 or the Phase 2 lists of acceptable carbohydrates
- ❖ Approximate time period is eight weeks
- ❖ BMI of 20 to 22

Category 2: The Adolescent Who Needs to Lose No Weight or Just a Few Pounds

To reiterate, this is the starting point for the nonoverweight teen. It will give your teenager a period of adjustment to a new way of eating, a way that does not rely on the nutritionally vacant calories of sugar. This adjustment needs to take place both physically and psychologically. At the beginning of this phase, your teen may feel a withdrawal period where they actually feel worse. This should last only one to three days at the most, depending on how addicted your child was to sugar or on how much sugar your child was in the habit of consuming.

In this category, I always recommend that my patients start at a carbohydrate level of 50 grams of complex carbohydrates in divided amounts at each meal. They may choose from the carbohydrates in the Phase 1 part of the diet or from the carbohydrates listed in Phase 2 of the diet. These will include beans, legumes, whole grains, and all vegetables.

SUMMARY OF PHASE 2, CATEGORY 2: THE HEALTH-CONSCIOUS TEEN

- ❖ All foods from Phase 1
- ❖ All beverages from Phase 1
- ❖ Complex carbohydrates in the amount of 50 grams per day in divided amounts per meal, chosen from those listed in Phase 1 or Phase 2
- ❖ Approximately four weeks in duration
- ❖ BMI of 20 to 22

The Next Generation Diet, Phase 2: *The Healthy Step—The General Rules*

THIS SECTION OF THE BOOK IS DESIGNED FOR PARENTS WITH CHILDREN of all ages. It will help define some of the foods that are now allowed in this phase of the diet.

As I've previously described, Phase 2 is the transition phase of the Next Generation Diet for those children who needed to lose weight. Phase 2 is also the beginning of the diet for those nonoverweight children whose parents want them to be healthy. This encompasses a broad range of children, hence, there are many similarities among the age groups.

In the last several chapters, I've discussed grams of carbohydrates, and now, to make things easier, I'd like to include a list of "kid friendly" foods and the amount of carbohydrates found in them. You want to be able to actually measure grams of carbohydrates, so you can either refer to this list, purchase a food-counter book from your local bookstore, or very carefully read the nutritional information label on the foods you buy.

❖ Carbohydrate Gram Counter ❖ for Kid Friendly Foods

Foods:	Grams of Carbohydrates
PROTEINS	
(includes any size serving of all fish, meat, poultry, and eggs)	0–trace
FATS	
any size serving of olive oil (or for that matter any oil)	0

CARBOHYDRATES

Vegetables

asparagus, 4 spears	2.6
bamboo shoots, ½ cup, cooked	4.0
green beans, ½ cup	3.9
broccoli, ½ cup, cooked	3.9
cauliflower, ½ cup, cooked	2.6
carrots, ½ cup, cooked	8.2
corn, ½ cup, cooked	20.6
peas, ½ cup, cooked	18.0
celery, ½ cup, diced, raw	2.2
lettuce, 1 head bibb	3.8
lettuce, 1 head iceberg	11.3
cucumber, ½ cup, sliced	1.4
onion, ½ cup, chopped	6.9
peppers, green or red, 1 medium	4.8
potato, ½ cup, diced, raw	13.5
yam, ½ cup, boiled	18.8
spinach, ½ cup, boiled	3.4

Fruits

apple, 2¾-inch diameter	21.0
apricots, 3 medium	11.8
cherry, ½ cup, pitted	11.3
strawberry, ½ cup, diced	5.2
watermelon, ½ cup, diced	5.7
cantaloupe, ½ cup	6.7
peach, 2½-inch diameter	9.7
grapefruit, Florida pink or red, 3¾-inch diameter	9.2

Milk
- whole, 8 ounces — 12.0
- soy, unsweetened, 8 ounces — 4.0

Cheese
- cheddar, 1 ounce — 0.6
- cottage, 1 cup — 7.0
- cream cheese, 1 ounce — 0.5
- Swiss, 1 ounce — 1.0
- Monterey jack, 1 ounce — 1.0
- mozzarella, 1 ounce — 0.5

Nuts and Seeds (all are 1-ounce serving)
- cashews — 8.0
- peanuts — 7.0
- walnuts — 3.0
- pecans — 5.0
- almonds — 6.0
- pistachios — 7.1
- pumpkin seeds — 15.3
- sunflower seeds — 6.0

Grains
- macaroni and cheese, ¾ cup — 34.0
- bagel, 3-inch round — 30.0
- muffin, corn — 20.0
- muffin, English, 4-inch round — 26.0
- waffles, 2, 4-inch square — 32.0
- oatmeal, 1 cup, cooked — 25.2
- popcorn, ½ ounce, popped — 8.0
- pretzels, 1 ounce — 22.5
- potato chips, 1 ounce — 16.0
- rice, brown, ½ cup, cooked — 26.0
- rice, white, ½ cup, cooked — 22.0

Sweets your child is used to eating
- chocolate milk shake, 8 ounces — 46.0
- ice cream sandwich, 4 ounces — 33.0
- orange juice, 6 ounces — 19.3
- orange soda, 12 ounces — 46.0
- cookie, 1 oatmeal — 18.0
- chocolate layer cake, ¹⁄₁₂ — 38.0
- Boston cream pie, ¹⁄₁₂ — 51.0
- granola bar, 6 ounces — 33.0
- chocolate pudding, ½ cup — 31.0
- rice pudding, ½ cup — 30.0

"gimme more" foods

For me, and ultimately for you, this is the fun part of the book because now you get to tell your kids what else they can eat.

Vegetables

Allowable vegetables now include carrots, peas, corn, winter squashes, parsnips, beets, and white potatoes. Sweet potatoes continue to be included in this phase of the diet. Just make sure that you are staying within the carbohydrate allowances.

Nuts and Seeds

Allowable nuts include almonds, pecans, macadamia nuts, walnuts, brazil nuts and peanuts. Your child is now allowed to have peanut butter, as long as it is sugar free and is made of nothing more than ground peanuts. These are the higher in protein and fat but lower in carbohydrate nuts. I allow 1 to 2 ounces per day of these. (Cashews and pistachios are not permitted in this phase of the diet because they are higher in carbohydrates.)

The seeds that are allowed include sunflower, pumpkin, and sesame. Your child can eat a total of 1 to 2 ounces per day of the permitted nuts *or* seeds.

Grains

This is the first phase of the diet where I allow grains, other than the small amount of brown rice allowed in Phase 1. I eliminate grains in Phase 1 to achieve a more significant weight loss. In Phase 2, where grains are allowed, I recommend the ones to which most people are the least sensitive. Those grains are buckwheat, kasha, millet, quinoa, amaranth, and teff. Note that grains that contain gluten are still *not* permitted, which means that breads and pasta made from routine grains are still not allowed in this phase. Gluten is the substance in certain flour products that makes the prebaked dough gooey. It is found in wheat, rye, and oat flours. In my experience, gluten has proven to be something to which many of my patients, especially children, have a food sensitivity. In the later chapters on health, I'll share many of the symptoms from which my patients have suffered, as well as their positive experiences when these allergenic substances were removed from their diet.

Legumes

Allowable legumes include lentils, kidney beans, black beans, lima beans, fava beans, black-eyed peas, and navy beans. Bean products such as tofu, tempeh, and seitan are also permitted.

These are the additional food products allowed in Phase 2, or the transition phase, of the diet. The amounts are not specified because it all comes down to counting carbohydrates, the amount of which will differ from child to child and from age to age. Once this phase is completed and your child is comfortable in this healthier nutritional environment, he or she is ready for Phase 3, or the Lifetime Phase, of the diet. This will begin in approximately one month for the nonoverweight child and two months for the overweight child, depending on their BMI (body mass index).

The Next Generation Diet, Phase 3: *A Lifetime of Healthy Eating*

O NCE YOUR CHILD HAS REACHED THIS POINT IN THE DIET—the forever stage—you deserve congratulations because now your child has become one of the healthiest kids on the block. All that's left for you to do is to ensure that this is something that can be maintained forever.

Phase 3 of the diet allows your child to eat protein, carbohydrates— both simple and complex—and simple sugars; but they must all be balanced. The ultimate purpose of this diet, and why it has so many long-lasting health benefits, is the regulation of insulin secretion and blood sugar levels. In order to do this, we must learn to properly balance our child's intake of food.

The tools you will need are the foods as I've described them in previous chapters, and the general rule you'll need to understand in order to successfully implement this new way of eating is really quite simple:

Each meal should contain 55 percent to 60 percent protein in the form of meats, fish, cheese, eggs, and nuts; 35 percent to 40 percent complex carbohydrates, such as those found in starchy vegetables, grains, legumes and beans, salad vegetables, and all other vegetables; and no more than 5 percent simple sugars, such as those found in milk, fruit, and other natural sweets.

Each meal should look something like this:

Figure 8   The Forever Diet

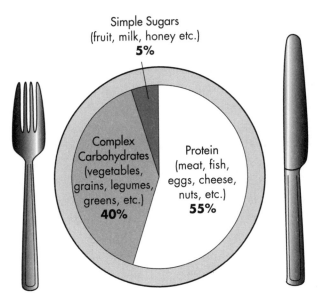

Simple Sugars
(fruit, milk, honey etc.)
5%

Complex
Carbohydrates
(vegetables,
grains, legumes,
greens, etc.)
40%

Protein
(meat, fish,
eggs, cheese,
nuts, etc.)
55%

the forever diet

This final phase of the diet is the way your children should be eating for the rest of their lives. It is a basic, healthy diet that incorporates all the important components of the available foods. No foods are eliminated, and in that respect I feel it is a much healthier and more balanced way of eating than a diet that is low in fat and high in carbohydrates. That diet is a diet of deprivation and is a very difficult one to maintain over the course of a lifetime. I have developed this diet to be relatively deprivation-free, so you and your child will be able to truly reap the benefits forever.

Essentially, in this forever phase of the diet, there is a one-step process for all members of the family. Once your child has entered this phase, there is no distinction made between those who have had to lose weight and those who began the diet, not to lose weight, but for health reasons. There is also no distinction among the three age groups, providing you follow the rule of balance and refer to the pie-plate diagram.

The food items that are now available on the diet are grains with gluten, breads, pastas, and other nuts. Also, at this point, simple sugars can be added to the diet in the form of fruit.

Grains

The grain products that can now be incorporated into your child's diet are grain products with glutens, including breads or bread-like products made with wheat, oats, rye, barley, and corn. Because of these additions, pasta can now be included in your child's diet. However, I prefer that it be made from artichoke flour, if possible, or rice flour, which had been available earlier on the diet.

Artichoke pasta is made from ground artichokes. Artichokes are a more complex carbohydrate and, therefore, form a healthier flour than the simple white flour that is used to make regular pasta. Rice pasta is healthier for the same reason.

There are many whole grain pastas available on the market today that I feel are much healthier products. Although the more common pastas are now allowed on the diet, I prefer my patients to look for the healthier ones.

Nuts

Nuts that are now allowed on the diet are pistachios and cashews. These nuts are higher in carbohydrates and should be saved for this phase of the diet.

Fruits

When it comes to snacks, I'm sure many people, even after reading the chapter on sugar, are still under the mistaken impression that all fruit is absolutely, 100 percent healthy. Let me remind you that this diet is a metabolically active one and that it will only work when all the components are working together simultaneously. In this diet, we are trying to regulate insulin secretion, thereby regulating blood sugar levels. This would be impossible to achieve without the elimination of fruit from the diet until this forever phase. Fruit is comprised in large part of a simple sugar, and it must be treated as such until we've corrected the metabolic imbalances present in your child's diet.

You and your child have reached this phase, so you've corrected all those metabolic imbalances. Your child can now start to include some fruit in his or her nutritional lifestyle program.

The truth is all fruits are not created equal. Your child should only eat fruit that contains the least amount of sugar per serving. These fruits are melons, including but not limited to honeydew, cantaloupe, crenshaw, and watermelon; berries, including but not limited to strawberries, blueberries, and raspberries. The next group of fruits most desirable in terms of their sugar ratio per serving include grapefruit, peaches, and plums.

As I've mentioned before, fruit juice is generally unacceptable at any stage of this diet. The reason is simple: in fruit juice the fiber, which allows the breakdown of the fruit by the body to occur more slowly, has been removed. If this is eliminated, then the fruit juice, something you've always been led to believe is infinitely healthy, is metabolized exactly the same way as a can of soda—and how many parents would like to see their child drink soda every morning for breakfast? Fruit juice contains a large amount of sugar to ingest at one time, and your child would have to eat a large amount of food to counterbalance that sugar load. This rule applies even to fresh squeezed juices that contain pulp from the fruit. There is not enough pulp to counter the effect of the amount of sugar from one glass of juice. Imagine trying to fit all the pulp from six oranges into that glass.

While we're on the subject of juice, it would only be fair to touch on the subject of vegetable juices. In general, vegetable juices are a far healthier product than fruit juices. I would suggest that the juice contain less than 15 percent of the sweeter vegetables, like carrots and beets. I allow my patients to use one carrot for flavor, and the rest of the juice should consist of green vegetables like broccoli, cucumber, and celery. Tomato juice is also acceptable in this phase of the diet. Fresh-squeezed is preferable to canned.

Other "free" foods on this phase of the diet include avocado and olives. Butter is also permitted, but margarine is never allowed, and I strongly warn against using it as a butter substitute. I also allow up to 4 ounces a day of yogurt in this stage of the diet, provided it is plain and unsweetened.

So there you have it. This diet can be infinitely rewarding in both the short and long run. Long term, it will correct the most common health problems prevalent in our children today. It does this by correcting the imbalances in the insulin and sugar regulatory mechanisms in your child's body. In the short term, you and your whole family will benefit by being able to eat a delicious, wholesome, balanced diet that really tastes good, while losing weight.

Happy eating!

How to Make the Diet Even More Successful

N<small>OW THAT YOU KNOW WHAT THE</small> N<small>EXT</small> G<small>ENERATION</small> D<small>IET</small> is all about, I would like to dispel some of the myths about diets in general, as well as introduce some of the general truths and helpful tips that will make dieting that much easier, with a higher chance of success.

top ten hints to a successful diet

The reason I believe diets are important for our children, both for those who are overweight and those who are not, is because most young people today are not making healthy eating choices. This puts them at risk for many short- and long-term health problems. For example, it has been shown that successful dieters maintain their reduced cholesterol levels and insulin levels after a five-year period if they manage to keep the weight off. This is exactly what we are trying to achieve—long-term success.

We can only accomplish this goal if we teach our children the skills necessary to practice healthy eating. The knowledge of what is healthy is not good enough. We have to give them an opportunity to practice healthy eating choices and make it fun in the process. I believe we can do both of these things.

Here are my top ten tips for a successful nutritional lifestyle plan:

1. *Never call an overweight child "fat."* Psychologists have found that children who are called fat begin to believe that it's an unalterable fact that they will remain that way, and therefore, more often than not, they fail at their attempts at dieting. The belief that one is fat, once it is established, almost never goes away. I know this from personal experience, as I still see a fat little boy staring back at me from the mirror. Instead, emphasize the possibility of regaining the trim physique that your child naturally had but lost.

2. *Try not to view your child's odd eating habits as a problem.* Often, children will go on strange tears where they only eat one type of food or foods of a particular color. As I've mentioned before, I once went on a diet that consisted entirely of french fries and chocolate pudding. After a while, the thrill of this wore off, and I was back to a regular diet, although not without successfully annoying my parents. My advice is to let them be, and it will pass. The more attention this behavior grabs, the more likely it is that it will last.

As a rule, overweight children are not good eaters. They just eat. Childhood food binges, food strikes, and other unusual habits are a normal part of a child's development. Children use the table as a stage for showing their independence, and food is often not the issue at all.

The eating process is one more way in which a child learns about the world. It's up to us to ensure that they learn the right things. Parents often forget or perhaps fail to realize the importance this plays in a child's development. I'll bet that if you sat back now for a few minutes and thought about your food habits as a child or what growing up in your household was like in its relationship to food, you'd be surprised at what you might come up with and the role these subtleties play in your life now. For example, I had a quirky habit of eating foods in a particular order from the dinner plate. I still do that. If you gave it some thought, I'm sure there are probably many of these eccentric habits you could name, too.

3. *Children learn from example.* They haven't yet developed all the mechanisms we use as adults to do what we don't want to do. They are unable to grasp the concept of "do as I say, not as I do." That's why we must set good examples that they can see. It is often easier for my young patients to be on a diet than it is for adults because they haven't yet learned the concept of rationalization. For the most part, they will still listen to what the doctor says, unless *you* sabotage it.

I have one patient named Ben. He has done very well on my program and follows the diet to the letter. Each time we have an appointment, he will bring me a list of foods that he would like to have. If I say no, he never asks again. His mother went on the diet about a year after Ben and one day they visited me together. She began to ask for different foods she would like to have, too. The only difference was that it was much more difficult to get her to accept the restrictions than it had been to get Ben to accept them. Later, he confided to me that his mother cheated more than he did, and boy, was he proud of that.

4. *Give a "five-minute warning."* Most of us have experienced the child who is too agitated to settle in for a meal, which results in the entire family's dinner being disrupted. For younger children, it's important to prepare them for meals by giving them what I call a five-minute warning, which will give them time enough to calm down in preparation for mealtime. Have them use the time to complete what they are doing, whether it's homework, watching TV, or playing outside. Have them go wash their hands and face, for instance. This will put a focus on mealtime as something that is taken very seriously, something that is a separate part of the day. In this way, eating will become equated with mealtime. It becomes something to think about and prepare for, and it starts to take on some meaning other than just a feeding. This particular point was very helpful for one girl named Kathy. She loved this aspect of mealtimes, and her mother told me how she

had incorporated this into her own playtimes with her friends and her dolls. Kathy, by the way, used to be a terribly picky and rambunctious child at the dinner table. Two weeks after this new behavior took firmly in the household, her conduct improved dramatically.

5. *Serve smaller meals more often.* Because overweight children are usually heavy snackers, I have found that they can live more easily with several smaller meals and still be able to lose weight. This will help keep blood sugar levels more or less constant, and it keeps the brain well supplied with the energy it requires. In the same way, eating the proper foods in this manner will prevent an overproduction of insulin. When either of these two things occur, one will begin to crave sugar and/or carbohydrates. Several smaller meals can help prevent this from occurring. This is almost never an issue while on the initial stages of this diet because food cravings and hunger are minimal.

By the same token, it may be necessary for some overweight children to have set times for eating. I only say this because overweight kids may think it is always appropriate to be eating, and, for long-term success, this may be a vital pattern or habit to establish.

The size of the portions you serve your child will obviously depend upon whether they are a large teenager or a small six-year-old. These guidelines were established in the chapters on diet and should be maintained. Suffice it to say, whatever your child's meal size may be, more frequently it should be a smaller portion. Setting portion controls for adults is much easier because we generally come in the same sizes. For children, it's different, and you, as a parent, have to be the best judge of proper portion size for your child.

6. *Take responsibility for the way your child eats.* It's easy if you remember this: children are the best of judge of *how much* they eat, and parents are the best judge of *what* they should eat. This is not always 100 percent accurate for the overweight child, but if you just changed what your overweight child ate (eliminating all sugars, for instance), even without changing the total amount of food eaten, you would be doing your child a tremendous service toward future health; and they would probably drop sev-

eral pounds in the process. Frequently, this happens to my patients in Phase 1 of the diet. Sometimes, when I've placed a child on the Next Generation Diet, the parents are in shock, and the only advice they follow is to remove white sugar from their child's diet, not to remove simple carbohydrates as well. They are amazed when they return to my office for their follow-up visit with a thinner kid.

7. *Make food "a close encounter of the healthy kind."* Good encounters with food at any age helps set the groundwork for sensible eating habits. It's impossible in this day and age to expect every meal to be a formal sit-down dinner, but even setting aside several meals a week for family dinner can make a world of difference in the character of what mealtimes look like in your household. This was always an important point in my house when I was growing up. Meals were an important time for the family to be together, and this has remained with me throughout my adult life.

8. *Never force your child to eat or encourage him or her to finish everything on the plate.* This only acts to set up a bad eating pattern. Better to keep the bigger picture in mind. Well-meaning parents and grandparents often think the worst if their child skips a meal or won't eat vegetables. The truth is, it's okay. Over time your child will get everything he or she needs to grow and develop normally. Your job is simply to offer healthful, nourishing meals on a daily basis with plenty of variety. If a child stops eating, it's usually because he or she is satisfied. Children, for the most part, will eat as much as they need to survive.

The pressure to eat everything on your plate, day after day, will only encourage a pattern of overeating or, worse yet, another type of eating disorder. I should know because this is what happened to me in my youth, and I strongly believe it's one of the reasons I grew up overweight. I never felt as if I were satisfying my parents unless all the food on my plate was gone. To this day, I find it next to impossible to leave food on my plate—that's how strongly these patterns become imprinted on us. I must put smaller amounts of food on my plate, otherwise it all gets eaten. As children, we want to satisfy our parents and make them proud of us. If they want us to eat everything on our plate, then that's what we do. Unfortunately, this may lead to eating patterns that are detrimental to our health. So don't worry if your kids skip meals.

9. *Don't make the dinner table a battlefield.* Avoid using those all-too-common phrases like "No dessert until you eat your vegetables" or "If you behave yourself at the dinner table, you can have a piece of candy." Food is food, and that's all it is. Don't give it any other connotation. We constantly have to be aware of whether we are using it as a reward or punishment. In the long run, food bribery creates far more problems than it solves. Besides, if you're anything like my parents, you will still wind up giving your child that dessert, whether they did what you wanted or not.

10. *Don't be a food tyrant.* Children, especially teenagers, will do anything to annoy their parents. Don't let them do this with food. Offer them their meals. If they want to eat it, they will. If not, they won't eat it. Don't ascribe more meaning to their behavior than it deserves.

Teenagers are especially prone to reacting badly to this kind of food terrorism. I can recall one such patient who was seriously acting out against his mother. Jeremy desperately wanted to lose weight, and because of this I thought dealing with him would be a walk in the park. He had nothing wrong with him other than a poor glucose tolerance test response curve, meaning he was hypoglycemic, an easily correctable problem with this diet. (As you may recall, hypoglycemia is the condition wherein your child's blood sugar will drop after eating sugar. Among other things, it can cause irritability and fatigue.) Jeremy's weight was fluctuating, but he was never really moving steadily in the right direction— down. Week after week, he would come into my office, always accompanied by his mother. Instinct told me that there was more here than met the eye. So finally, I decided to interview him without his mother present, which is something I often do with my teenage patients. He told me that his mom was "always on my case." She was constantly telling him every step of the way what he should and should not be doing. He was resenting her and resenting the diet, and for this reason he was doomed for failure. I then asked Jeremy if I could speak privately to his mother. Reluctantly, he agreed. I explained to her the concept of "food tyrant." She immediately got what I meant and, with much effort on her part, was able to adjust her behavior, allowing Jeremy to lose the weight he wanted.

bonus tip

11. *Only buy the foods you want your child to eat and allow them to make their own choices from this selection.* It's up to you as parents, to supply your children with the types of foods that they need to become good eaters. Yes, it's true that your child is able to buy their own foods at school, without your guidance, but by setting the proper tone, without becoming overbearing, it will allow your teenagers to make the *right* decisions. Our faith in them will ultimately empower them into doing the right thing. It's no different from teaching them the right way to behave. We are not with them 100 percent of the time, yet we expect them to behave just as appropriately when we're not around as when we are. This is an expectation we build into our relationship with our children. The same holds for food. I can't stress strongly enough that eating is a *learned* behavior, just like any other. Unfortunately, we don't treat it as such, and if we are to succeed in making our children healthier, we must do just that.

Try not to let your child feel deprived. The key is to emphasize that what they are now eating is better for them. Set a good example by eating the right foods yourself. That's why I've tried to explain the health benefits of the Next Generation Diet. It's important that you become convinced of the merits of this diet so that you can be an effective coach for your child. Your child will only be as good on this diet as you allow him or her to be. So, give them the space to make it happen. It may take some time, but it's well worth the effort.

❖ The Golden Rules of the Next Generation Diet ❖

- ❖ Avoid sugar or simple carbohydrates in any form (White bread and white pasta are in effect sugar.)
- ❖ Avoid fruit juice, soda, and milk.
- ❖ Incorporate some fats into your child's diet—they are not all bad.
- ❖ Remember portion control—and balance, balance, balance.
- ❖ Eat organically whenever possible.
- ❖ Exercise is crucial.
- ❖ All children should avoid alcohol and caffeine.
- ❖ Make mealtimes activities unto themselves—family time.
- ❖ Never skip meals.
- ❖ Avoid processed foods whenever possible.
- ❖ Read nutrition labels very carefully (look for sugars in all their disguises, trans fats, and other unhealthy things).

the Health Connection: How *to* Prevent Disease

Your Child's Health

17

$\mathbf{D}$ARLA WAS FIFTEEN YEARS OLD. Her mother brought her to me because she was having bimonthly periods. She was also anemic and, as a result, suffered from constant fatigue. Her mother was frightened to death because her gynecologist wanted the girl to take birth control pills. Neither mother nor daughter was particularly keen on this solution. Yet this is a common answer to many female menstrual irregularities. I can't tell you how many adult patients I see because their gynecologist has put them on birth control pills, with the result being that they can't seem to lose any weight and, in fact, have gained weight since starting the medication.

After viewing the results of a thorough history and physical examination, routine blood tests, a glucose tolerance test, and a cytotoxic food sensitivity test, I placed Darla on a yeast-free, Phase 1 diet and eliminated all of her food allergies. I also provided her with several nutritional supplements, like boron, genestein (which is a soy derivative), folic acid, caprylic acid, and mycocidin.

In just two short months, Darla's menstrual cycle went back to normal, and in the process, she lost 17 pounds.

In overweight boys and girls, excess weight can cause developmental problems of puberty. Estrogen is stored in adipose tissue, so you can expect to see menstrual irregularities in young girls and the delay of secondary sexual characteristics in young boys, such as the development of pubic, underarm, and facial air, the deepening of the voice, the widening of the chest, and the development of more lean muscle mass and increased muscle tone.

diet and health

By this time you should understand that your child's (and your) health is inextricably tied to diet. How could it not be? Everything your child eats or drinks becomes a part of him or her in one way or another. The body's building blocks come from the diet, and if the right building blocks are not supplied, the child cannot grow to be a healthy, vibrant adult.

But in addition to eating well, there are some natural and complementary medical approaches that I recommend to deal with many of the most common childhood complaints. Complementary medicine is ideally suited for this purpose because it combines the best of all medical worlds in its aim to achieve universal health.

Jason, who was twelve years old, was brought to me because he suffered from asthma as well as a variety of other allergies. Even before examining him closely, I could see he was between 10 and 15 pounds overweight. I familiarized myself thoroughly with his medical history, then gave him a physical examination, including routine blood tests.

Knowing that there can often be a strong relationship between nutrition, obesity, and asthma, I also conducted a cytotoxic food sensitivity test, which systematically tests the blood against fifty or so of the most common food allergens. This test showed Jason to be highly sensitive to all grains, except rice, and to have a candida sensitivity. Because of the latter sensitivity, I needed to remove all sugars and anything from his diet that contained yeast. This meant breads, most cheeses, and vinegar. (Later in this book, I will be explaining more about those individuals who need a yeast-restricted diet, along with some of the symptoms your child may be experiencing if he or she has a yeast problem.)

By placing Jason on Phase 1, sugars were easily eliminated from his diet. I believe there is a correlation between the increase in sugar consumption and the increase in the incidence of such childhood diseases as asthma, allergies, and attention deficit disorder.

Within a matter of a couple of days of going on the diet, Jason began losing weight. As a result, he had a tremendous gain in energy, and his school performance improved markedly. But, more importantly, his allergies began to clear up, and for the first time in his life, he was able to forgo his asthma medication. I believe the reason his allergies and asthma symptoms may have begun to fade so quickly was due to the immediate elimination of gluten and milk from his diet. These substances are the source of many food sensitivities in my patients. The elimination of yeast and sugar takes longer to produce a positive effect. The Next Generation Diet eliminated all these food items, and the result was not only weight loss, but improved health.

if it ain't broke, don't fix it

Jason's parents were so impressed by the changes in their son that they approached me and asked if I could help their other child, Jeffrey. Jeffrey was a year older than Jason and was having some minor behavioral problems at school. He was becoming forgetful, unwilling to participate in class, and unwilling to do his homework, and, upon coming home from school in the afternoon, he always insisted on taking a nap. Of all the things his parents were concerned about, this was the most troubling because Jeffrey had always been such an active child and now all he wanted to do was sleep. They had already taken him to several doctors, so they knew there were no physical abnormalities that could be detected by routine testing.

There was one crucial difference between the two boys. Whereas Jason was built like his mother, short and stocky, Jeffrey was built more like his father, tall and lean. Because of these differences, Jeffrey's parents couldn't understand what could possibly be wrong with the way their oldest son ate, and so they were skeptical that an improper diet might be at the heart of the problem. "He's so thin," they kept saying. "How could his diet possibly have anything to do with his allergies?" This is a common refrain. Parents often regard their children's health with the attitude of, "If it ain't broke, don't fix it." Of course, this is nonsense. For one thing, in regard to putting on weight, some children have a higher metabolism that acts to keep the weight off. However, this doesn't mean that the foods they're eating are good for them. Secondly, as I've stated before, eating habits are learned early in life, and metabolic rates change as we get older. The child who can (and does) eat everything without gaining a pound may well turn into the adult who eats everything and accumulates pounds at an alarming rate.

As part of my examination of Jeffrey, I performed a glucose tolerance test, routine chemistries, and a food sensitivity test. The results were very much the same as they were with Jason, and so I removed all simple sugars from his diet by placing him on Phase 2 of the diet and also removed anything that contained yeast.

In less than three weeks, the changes in Jeffrey were quite evident. His allergies virtually disappeared, and his ability to concentrate was markedly improved. In addition, his behavior at school had improved so much that his parents had received a call from the administration because his teachers could not believe he was the same boy who'd made so much trouble only weeks before. He was much calmer and easier to get along with. The diet corrected the gross imbalances in Jeffrey's glucose tolerance curve. The simple corrections in his diet made a world of difference in his life.

Not unsurprisingly, his parents were amazed at the changes in their son because they thought there was nothing wrong with the way Jeffrey ate. They could not believe that food played such a major role in his life.

a personal note

I have not eaten fast food in thirteen years. The only reason I can give for this is that I never acquired a taste for it when I was a child. It is the one thing my parents did properly, in terms of eating habits. I was a child of the television generation, so I was constantly bombarded with messages to eat at the fast food chains. I would beg to eat there, but my parents were adamantly against it. I only began to eat there as a young adult, while I was away at college. The thrill of doing this to defy my parents wore off rather quickly. I would never even think of going to one of those places today, in large part because that pattern had not been set early in life.

Every day, adult patients come to me, and in preparation for writing this book, I have made it a point to quiz them about the types of foods they ate as a child, including their likes and dislikes. Invariably, the types of foods they enjoy as adults are exactly the kinds of foods they enjoyed as a child, and most importantly, the foods they most loved as a child are the foods they will return to when they need comforting, the so-called comfort foods. We all have them. Mine include pasta and ice cream. One of the treats I enjoyed as a child was Carvel ice cream. To this day, every time I walk or drive past a Carvel, like Pavlov's dog, I begin to salivate and I have an almost overwhelming urge to stop. This only illustrates the powerful influence our childhood experiences exert on our adult lives. And, as a parent, you must be aware of the tremendous power you have to help shape the nutritional habits of your children.

the tide is turning

There's never been a time in our history when so many children are suffering from chronic illnesses — illnesses that we would expect to see in adults, like diabetes, hypertension, and high cholesterol. There is also an alarming increase in the number of children suffering from asthma and allergies. However, what I think is an even more disturbing fact is that children are suffering from ever more learning disabilities, including attention deficit hyperactivity disorder and behavioral problems in school.

It's true that at the turn of the century, there were infectious diseases that ran rampant and the infant mortality rate was quite high. But today we live in the age of antibiotics, which have been able to cure most of the infectious diseases that affect our part of the world. But with the advent of these wonder drugs, a disturbing question arises. Could these antibiotics, at the same time they have worked wonders in curing many infectious diseases, be causing others?

No one knows the answer for sure, but I believe that it may play a role. And I also believe that the overprescription of antibiotics in the pediatric population is of serious concern. I am not alone in that belief. Recently, a growing number of conventional doctors are beginning to publish articles on the subject of the potentially dangerous overuse of antibiotics. In one study, for instance, I was amazed to read that several physicians interviewed admitted that even though they knew that their patient was infected with a virus as the cause of their upper respiratory infection, they still prescribed an antibiotic because they believed that if they didn't they would feel guilty for not prescribing something. It should be noted — and underscored — that antibiotics are not effective against viruses. It's also true that most patients, when they visit a doctor, expect to walk out of the office with a prescription in hand; and if the doctor doesn't give it to them, then the patient often feels as if he or she did not have a productive visit. It's certainly worth investigating the repercussions of such indiscriminate overprescription of very expensive and potentially very toxic medications, which, in many cases, may not be necessary.

Many bacteria are becoming increasingly resistant to even the most sophisticated antibiotics, and it is the doctor's responsibility not to haphazardly prescribe antibiotics. At the same time, it is the patient's responsibility not to demand the newest antibiotic on the market. In the long run, not only will this save us financially, but more importantly it will protect us from so called "super-bacteria" to which we have built up no resistance and for which there is no cure.

Certainly, there are illnesses that call for prescription drugs, and that is why I practice complementary or integrative medicine, so I can use the best of all worlds to treat my patients. But just as certainly, there are natural ways to deal with disease, as well as simple and natural ways to *prevent* disease, which is surely the more desired solution.

With this in mind, it shouldn't be much of a stretch to believe that the way your child eats also affects his or her health, whether or not he or she suffers from a weight problem.

In the next few chapters, we will take a look at some of the most common childhood health problems, their connection to diet, and the ways I try to deal with them in my practice. Besides all the cardiovascular problems, there are orthopedic abnormalities, such as knee and joint pains that often require arthroscopic surgery; hypoventilation (shortness of breath); endocrinopathies, such as thyroid disease and premature onset of puberty; and skin problems, such as acne, ezcema, and psoriasis. Whatever your own child's problem, be aware that in addition to your pediatrician's care and the program offered in this book, there may be other alternative or complementary solutions to your child's health problems.

18

The
Insulin Factor
and Diabetes

L ET'S LOOK AT THE CHILD WHO EATS CANDY ALL DAY LONG, as was the case of a young girl I observed recently while waiting at an airport for a delayed flight. I began watching a family sitting not far from me. There were four children, all slightly overweight. But one girl was obese. In her hand was the largest bag of candy I'd ever seen. During the course of the next couple of hours, she proceeded to eat the entire contents of the bag. This meant that her insulin level was continuously elevated for that entire time, as her body tried to metabolize the sugar load she was placing on her system. This does not just apply to candy. Let's remember that simple carbohydrates are metabolized in the body in the same way sugar is. For instance, if the girl were to have a smaller bag of candy followed by a bag of pretzels, it would still have the same effect on her body and her metabolism. She could even have substituted a piece of fruit for either the candy or the pretzels, and the same thing would have happened.

The Next Generation Diet is a healthy diet because it helps balance your child's blood sugar and insulin levels. Because the typical American diet is high in sugar, and because insulin is secreted in the body as a result of the ingestion of sugar (or any food, for that matter), the typical American diet is also high in insulin.

The fundamental problem with sugar or any other simple carbohydrate is the rapidity with which it is absorbed and digested. Insulin, which is the storage hormone for the body, may do its job of bringing the blood sugar back down with too much efficiency, and as a result, your child's blood sugar level may fall too rapidly, leading to hypoglycemia, or low blood sugar. These symptoms range from dizziness and fatigue to crying spells, irritability, aggression, depression, and moodiness.

When your child's body takes in a sugar load, whether in the form of white sugar or simple carbohydrates, there can be four responses:

1. Normal
2. Borderline hypoglycemia
3. Hypoglycemia
4. Diabetes

Please refer to the graphs in Chapter 4 for a more detailed explanation and a refresher on what these states are.

A glucose tolerance test is something I perform on about 90 percent of my patients. There is a good deal of information that can be obtained from this very simple test. As I've explained earlier, it is a series of blood tests in which the blood sugar is monitored at various time intervals for up to six hours after the ingestion of a specific amount of glucose, determined by the weight of the patient.

why worry about insulin? my child's not diabetic.

The long-term consequences of an imbalance in the insulin and blood sugar levels can lead to, among other things, heart disease, diabetes, and high blood pressure. The association between obesity and diabetes mellitus and cardiovascular risk is thought to be partially mediated by insulin.

Let me explain this a little further. Over time, there is a direct relationship between insulin levels and disease. This means that when there is an increased amount of insulin in the body, the risk of disease increases. If your child's body were constantly metabolizing sugars or simple carbohydrates, it would result in increased circulating levels of insulin.

Insulin resistance is yet another issue thought to play a role in overall, long-term health. Insulin resistance is the mechanism whereby the receptors in the body become less sensitive to the insulin that is being secreted. This means that your child's body will have to produce more insulin to get the same effect, and some of the receptors may just stop working. For example, during a glucose tolerance test, your child's blood sugar will rise to 130 to 170. In a normal child, the amount of insulin that is needed to bring this blood sugar back down to a normal range is approximately 45 units. In a child with insulin resistance, the amount of insulin needed to cause this same response is 60 or greater.

Therefore, your child's body will have to produce extra insulin to bring down the blood sugar level. However, in children, it is still unclear as to whether increased circulating levels of insulin or the presence of insulin resistance is the primary problem in the cause of the increase of these diseases. Eventually, the combination of a high glucose load (the typical American diet) and the high insulin demand may wear out your child's pancreas, which may then fail to secrete the necessary amounts of insulin.

Insulin levels are directly related to increases in body fatness, particularly in those who tend to collect fat around the middle. This means that the heavier you are, the more insulin the body requires to bring your blood sugar down to the normal range. The combination of increased insulin and insulin resistance (and in severe cases, followed by failure to produce insulin) is the mechanism responsible for non-insulin-dependent, or type II, diabetes mellitus, a disease whose increase closely parallels the increased prevalence of obesity. Traditionally, this is not a disease that generally affects children. Most diabetic children are insulin-dependent type I diabetics, and their bodies simply do not produce insulin at all.

However, in the July 1997 issue of the medical journal *Pediatrics*, researchers reported that they found a dramatic increase in the incidence of type II diabetes among young patients.

In this study, nearly all the children with type II diabetes were obese, and more than 30 percent had high blood pressure. Type II diabetes, "once believed to be a disease of predominantly obese adults, is on the rise in the pediatric population," the researchers wrote. The study indicated that many American children eat too much and are overweight, said Dr. Gerald Bernstein, president-elect of the American Diabetes Association. "What this opens the door to is, one, we have to undergo a major cultural adjustment to food and exercise. Two, routine screening in pediatric offices should be incorporated into the care of children who are high-risk."

I could not agree more with this statement. We need to redefine the dietary habits of our children. I am hoping this book will help you, as parents, make that cultural adjustment we so desperately need. The longer your child is overweight, the greater the likelihood is that he or she will develop diabetes, even as a child, not just as an adult. This is not to say that nonoverweight adults do not develop diabetes. They do, all the time. However, whether they are thin or obese, the mechanism by which they develop the type II diabetes is usually the same, insulin resistance. Therefore, don't make the mistake of thinking that your nonoverweight child is safe. Make the Next Generation Diet important for all your children—whether they are overweight or not.

Understanding Obesity in Youth—A Statement for Healthcare Professionals, from the Committee on Atherosclerosis and Hypertension in the Young of the Council on Cardiovascular Disease in the Young, and the Nutrition Committee of the American Heart Association, is a multipage statement discussing the swift rise in obesity in our children and some of the health implications associated with this. After years of research, we are beginning to realize that the harm we cause our bodies when we are young does take its toll on us as adults.

diabetes mellitus

I have already mentioned diabetes mellitus as the premier diet-related disorder plaguing our country today. This is a disease that affects millions of people around the world. It is a disorder of the body's ability to process foods that are eaten, especially sugars and simple carbohydrates, leading to an excess of blood sugar.

This disease lasts a lifetime. It is not curable, so it is a condition with which one must learn to live. There are many complications to this disease, including heart disease, peripheral vascular disease, eye and vision problems, kidney disease, and high blood pressure, to name a few.

There are two types of diabetes mellitus: (1) juvenile onset or type I, which is also known as insulin-dependent because the body has lost its ability either to produce insulin or to utilize the insulin that was produced; and (2) adult onset or type II, which is also known as non-insulin-dependent because the body could still produce insulin, but the insulin was not being used, a condition known as insulin resistance.

Traditional wisdom was always that children had type I diabetes and required insulin, and adults had type II and could hopefully control the disease with diet or oral hypoglycemic medications, or a combination of the two. The delineation is no longer so simple. Type II diabetes is generally caused by being overweight. Because of the marked rise in obesity in our youth, type II diabetes is rapidly rising in the pediatric population. Because of the long-standing obesity problem in the adult population, more and more adults are finding it necessary to use insulin.

The Next Generation Diet can be safely used for the overweight child who has developed type II diabetes. I also feel it can be successfully used to avoid this dreaded disease, if the diet is begun early enough. However, in the two situations I've just outlined, medications usually need to be adjusted, and I would not suggest you attempt to do this without the help of a physician. I have used this diet successfully in many patients. But I am very reluctant to advise you in a book on how to do this on your own. Diabetes is a very serious illness and must be treated very cautiously.

If you do try this on your own, do so on a trial basis and monitor your child's blood sugar very carefully. And please remember, if in doubt, err on the side of caution and consult your pediatrician.

There are many nutritional supplements that can help control your child's blood sugar. These include chromium picolinate, vanadyl sulfate, thiotic acid, biotin, and zinc, to name a few.

Diabetes Mellitus Treatment, in Short

❖ Phase 1 diet
❖ Nutritional supplementation, as described above

Syndrome X

I HAVE TREATED ONE CHILD WITH HIGH BLOOD PRESSURE. His name was Brian, he was fourteen years old, and he was not overweight. In fact, he was in such great shape and so good an athlete that he was the captain of his junior high school basketball team. Of late, he had not been feeling well. He was getting headaches, and his normal stamina was way down. His worried parents took him to their local pediatrician who diagnosed Brian as having hypertension and wanted to place the young man on medication. His parents were despondent over this diagnosis and were quite concerned that he would die of a heart attack on the court, like other young kids have today. At the same time, they were frightened by the approach of conventional physicians, which was to immediately place Brian on medication that was made for adults. As with most parents, they did not want to see their child on medication for the rest of his life, if it could be at all avoided. Yet naturally, they could not stand by and do nothing for their child.

I believed their instinct to avoid medication was correct. There are many reasons why you would not want your child on adult high blood pressure medication for life. The first reason is that these medications were not intended to be used on people continuously over the course of fifty, sixty, or even seventy years. Secondly, teenage girls or young women of reproductive age should never be given certain medications for fear of the effect they would have if they were to become pregnant. Thirdly, a diagnosis of hypertension will have a decided effect on a teenager's ability to obtain health and life insurance. In fact, there's a good chance a child so diagnosed will be doomed to a lifetime of not having adequate medical coverage.

After hearing their story, I believed I might be able to do something for Brian, and I convinced his parents to let me examine him. First, I ran a glucose tolerance test on him, as well as insulin levels. I also ran another battery of tests, including food sensitivities. Sure enough, as I suspected, Brian's insulin levels were sky-high, and his glucose tolerance test was vastly abnormal. In fact, his insulin level was three times normal and, as a result of this, he became extremely hypoglycemic after eating a meal high in glucose. Other abnormalities on his blood profiles were high triglycerides and, for an athlete, a low HDL cholesterol level (the "good" cholesterol).

When I asked his parents what they were feeding their child, they replied, "Oh, you know, the usual things kids eat—candy after school, fruit juice throughout the day, fruit as snacks, as well as soda with dinner." Fast food was a twice weekly ritual for the family, and breakfast was a cereal loaded with sugar, drowning in milk.

I was surprised Brian could function at all. He was normally consuming more glucose at each meal and as snacks than I had given him with the glucose tolerance test. Because the cornerstone of my diet involves banning the intake of sugar, I immediately removed all processed and refined sugar from his diet and placed him on the Phase 2 diet. By doing this, I was able to correct the insulin imbalance that drove his blood pressure so high. I also placed him on a host of nutritional supplements which included chromium polynicotinate and vanadyl sulfate to correct his sugar imbalance and magnesium to correct his high blood pressure. (See Chapter 26 for a discussion of nutritional supplements.) Within two weeks, Brian's blood pressure responded positively. His pediatrician conducted another physical examination and couldn't believe that Brian's blood pressure was back to normal. Not only that, but his energy returned, and he was playing ball better than ever. Two months after our initial consultation, I redid Brian's blood work, and his insulin levels had returned to normal, as had his triglycerides. His HDL cholesterol level had also improved.

Now, four years later, Brian's blood pressure remains well within the normal range. He has not required any medication and has continued to take his supplements, and he just won a basketball scholarship to college.

CHAOS

Brian was a clear example of what is now called Syndrome X, so named because medicine is unsure of some of the aspects of this condition. However, it is becoming increasingly clear that many of the most common American health hazards may be part of this same process.

CHAOS is an acronym standing for the related disorders of this syndrome: *C*oronary heart disease, *H*ypertension and dyslipidemia, *A*dult-onset diabetes (remember, this is becoming more and more prevalent in children), *O*besity, and *S*troke.

Dyslipidemia is the term for an imbalance in the lipid blood profile. The lipid blood profile includes cholesterol (HDL and LDL) and triglycerides. In someone with dyslipidemia, the usual pattern is an elevated triglyceride level (greater than 150, although I define it as greater than 100) and a low HDL cholesterol (under 45 for girls and under 35 for boys).

Coronary heart disease is actually atherosclerosis, or clogged arteries. If you think this doesn't happen to children, just wait until the next chapter when I'll present strong evidence to the contrary.

Syndrome X evolves from insulin resistance and the resulting *hyper-insulinism*, the medical term for too much insulin in the bloodstream. You will remember that this resistance comes from having consumed too much sugar in the diet over the course of time. This chronic sugar load results in a constant demand on the pancreas to secrete insulin to bring your child's blood sugar back to the normal range. The insulin will also cause the conversion of some of the glucose to glycogen for immediate energy, and some of the glucose will be brought to the liver, converted to triglycerides and then stored as fat. The tissues that do all this eventually become fatigued from being activated at all times, and as a result, your child's body will need more and more insulin to do the same job.

According to David Moeller, M.D., of the Harvard Medical School, it appears that 20 percent of all Americans are as resistant to insulin as diabetics are. By the same token, roughly 25 percent of the population, or 60 million people (many of them children), especially if they are overweight, are sensitive to carbohydrates. This means that when they eat excess carbohydrates, even whole grains, they will get a glucose and insulin overload in the bloodstream.

Risk Factors for Syndrome X

1. Overweight individuals have a much greater risk of insulin resistance than do those who are lean.

2. A sedentary lifestyle and lack of muscle mass contributes to insulin resistance.

3. Certain drugs, such as Beta blockers and diuretics, and tobacco.

4. Hypertension.

Hypertension

Hypertension is becoming increasingly prevalent in the childhood years, and it may have its origin in Syndrome X.

Increased insulin levels in the bloodstream can result in the increased release of other hormones. Some of these hormones may be part of the sympathetic nervous system, leading to an increased release of catecholamines, or corticosteroids.

Corticosteroids are the substances produced by the body in the fight-or-flight reaction, which causes an increase in blood pressure so you can avoid predators. This reaction was never meant to occur on an ongoing basis. It appears that sugar, and in turn the resulting oversecretion of insulin, may be causing these corticosteroids to be hypersecreted and thus be in abundance in your child's blood. Because there are few true fight-or-flight situations nowadays, this reaction occurs in other stressful situations in which we find ourselves, such as being stuck in traffic jams, waiting for late buses, worrying about taking tests or doing homework, and the like.

Norepinephrine, which is one of the corticosteroids, along with the excess insulin, can also lead to renal sodium (salt) and fluid retention, which in turn affects the kidneys, which some researchers believe leads to high blood pressure.

In a study published in the *Journal of the American Medical Association,* it was found that children of people who experience early cardiovascular disease were much more likely to be obese and to develop future cardiovascular disease in early adulthood. This occurred in children as young as five whose parents had heart problems prior to the age of fifty.

The findings suggested that early obesity appears to bring on the "premature onset of other risk factors," according to an editorial in the *Journal.* These other risk factors are high cholesterol, high blood pressure, hypoglycemia, or diabetes. Linda Van Horn and Dr. Philip Greeland, authors of the editorial and professors of preventive medicine at Northwestern University Medical School, wrote, "This study underscores the importance of primary prevention of coronary artery disease beginning in childhood."

There are many supplements that could help in the treatment of Syndrome X and for the treatment of the individual parts of this disease. For the management of hypertension, I use magnesium, garlic, taurine, cayenne, coenzyme Q10, and the omega-3 fatty acids. The doses must be specific for each patient, and therefore I recommend you see a doctor who is familiar with complementary medicine if you wish to use these supplements.

Hypertension Treatment in Short

❖ Phase 1 or Phase 2 diet, as appropriate

❖ Nutritional supplementation as outlined above

Syndrome X can strike any of your children, and it is known in medical circles as the "silent killer," not usually manifesting itself until there is hypertension or diabetes. Too few physicians are aware of Syndrome X, and therefore they will not be able to guide you properly. I encourage you to ask your child's physician about this if your child has any of the symptoms or blood markers for this dreaded syndrome.

The Great Cholesterol Debate

J ENNIFER CAME TO SEE ME WITH A WEIGHT PROBLEM. The first thing her parents told me was that Jenn, who was fifteen, was a very finicky eater who did not like many foods. I thought to myself, somewhat incredulously, as Jennifer was about 25 pounds overweight, that there had to be something going on here that had yet to reveal itself. After all, Jennifer did not become 25 pounds overweight simply by not eating.

During her initial workup, blood work was taken, along with a glucose tolerance test. These tests showed a markedly abnormal glucose tolerance, markedly increased insulin levels, and a cholesterol count of 270, with an HDL of 41 and triglycerides of 330.

These figures would constitute a disaster for anybody's blood chemistry profile, but what made this even more significant was that Jennifer was so young. In fact, this was a blood chemistry you would expect to find in a sixty-year-old man who is 30 to 50 pounds overweight, drinks, smokes, and has just suffered his first heart attack. Jennifer's cholesterol should have been somewhere between 160 and 190. Her HDL should have been between 50 and 60, and her triglycerides should have been no more than 100. These alarming numbers placed Jennifer well above average risk for cardiovascular disease.

Usually, women (young and through menopause) are protected from cardiovascular disease by the beneficial effects of estrogen, but obviously this was not the case with Jennifer. I immediately placed her on the Phase 1 diet, which consisted of drastically lowering the amount of carbohydrates she ate, as well as eliminating sugar in any form (including fruit, bread, and sugar in all its usual disguises). She was allowed to eat foods that many would consider high in fat and cholesterol, like eggs for breakfast and cheeseburgers for lunch. I also permitted her to have bacon, peanut butter, cream cheese, and other foods that do not look as if they should be on a weight-loss diet, let alone a diet that is designed to bring down your cholesterol.

I also placed Jennifer on certain nutritional supplements, which, in my clinical experience, have proven to help in regulating a lipid problem. These included lecithin, pantethine, and the omega-3 fatty acids, found in fish oils. I would also use GLA, an omega-6 fatty acid, in this instance.

Before visiting my office, I often have prospective patients prepare a food diary. Jennifer was no exception. I reviewed her food diary and found that the only foods this child would eat were various kinds of candy, ice cream twice a day, pizza, and a cereal loaded with sugar. No matter how hard they tried, this was all her parents could get her to eat.

Clearly, there was some sort of emotional struggle going on, and I knew that, because of the potential psychological ramifications, I had to tread very lightly. And so, what we did was to experiment to see if we could change some of these deadly dietary patterns that had, unfortunately, taken firm root. I gave her mother a two-week diet plan, similar to the one you'll find in this book, and asked her not to deviate one bit, even if it meant that her daughter might go to bed without any supper. I assured her that her child would not starve. Often, food is used as a weapon both by the child and the parent. Children will eat when they need to. It is a simple human trait, genetically programmed into us. Unless there is a true, serious psychological problem or a political statement to be made, no one will voluntarily starve to death.

At the end of the two-week period, her mother reported to me that despite the fact that it was not a pleasant experience for the family, she had done what I'd asked. Jennifer had maintained the diet and had taken the nutritional supplements I had recommended. Resistance was high, and yet, by the ninth day, Jennifer had begun to eat what was given to her. When I questioned her, she actually admitted that she was beginning to like vegetables, which only proved my point: your child's dietary habits will only be as good as you allow them to be.

In the next four weeks, Jennifer not only lost 20 pounds, but her blood results showed a marked improvement: her cholesterol level was 188; her HDL count 72, and her triglycerides had fallen to an astonishing 48.

Needless to say, her parents were stunned. The diet she was eating flew in the face of convention and the food pyramid that is ingrained into every child in school.

Quietly, with a tear of relief in her eye, Jennifer thanked me, and I could see that she was going to be okay. Today, because she has maintained this diet, she is at her goal weight, with perfect blood chemistries.

determining risk for heart disease

This is how medical science makes a risk determination—you are either above, at, or below average for cardiovascular disease, depending on the ratios of certain numbers. To get this number, you simply divide the total cholesterol by the HDL and you will get a ratio. Ideally, this number should be below 4.0. Another ratio that I look at that most physicians ignore is the ratio of triglycerides to HDL.

In a study led by Dr. J. Michael Gaziano of the Brigham and Women's Hospital in Boston, it was found that the ratio of triglycerides to HDL was the strongest predictor of a heart attack, even more accurate than the usual total cholesterol-HDL ratio many physicians use. In the study, published in *Circulation*, there was a sixteen-fold increased risk for heart attack associated with an increased triglyceride level and a decreased HDL level. Triglycerides are much easier to control by diet and exercise. The Next Generation Diet, low in sugars and high in omega-3 fatty acids, can significantly lower your child's triglyceride levels, hence their cardiovascular risk.

Recently, the medical community has taken a marked interest in a cardiac risk factor called *homocysteine* which is an intermediary amino acid produced by our bodies when it converts methionine to lysine. The homocysteine level can rise when the body loses its ability to complete this conversion due to a lack of B vitamins and other enzymes; the process is still not completely understood. Homocysteine is proving to be a better indicator of coronary artery disease in adults than what I've been describing to you. It is an indicator I have routinely used in my adult patients for years now. However, there have been no studies so far to indicate its usefulness in the pediatric population, so it is not something I routinely measure in my patients who are children.

when does heart disease begin?

At what age do you think cholesterol problems begin to occur? Forty? Fifty? Even sixty years old? Absolutely not. High cholesterol and the health problems associated with it don't just appear spontaneously when we reach adulthood. Like so many other things, this is fast becoming a problem of childhood, and it is now being recognized as beginning in childhood.

Today we know that high cholesterol is a problem of many young adults, and, amazingly enough, it is thought to have its onset when a child is as young as six years old. This was only recently discovered when, twenty-five years ago, after the end of the Vietnam War, autopsies were conducted on soldiers who perished there. In the eighteen- and nineteen-year-old soldiers who had been killed, autopsies showed atherosclerotic cardiovascular disease, or hardening of the arteries. Cholesterol plaques had already begun to form in these young adults. Because these plaques were present at autopsy, this meant they had been there for at least several years, which in turn told researchers that the plaques had begun to form in these young men as early as when they were twelve years old.

It was assumed that the results were due to a childhood diet high in fat. I disagree. Instead, I believe it was the combination of a diet that had an emphasis both on refined sugars and carbohydrates.

High Blood Cholesterol/Triglyceride Treatment in Short

❖ Phase 1 or Phase 2 diet, as appropriate
❖ Nutritional supplements that include lecithin, pantethine, and omega-3 fatty acids

fast but wrong food

You were probably wondering when I was going to discuss the issue of fast food. Well, here it is. As you might imagine, I don't think very highly of it. I do understand, however, that for many Americans it is a necessary evil. So, instead of saying, "Don't feed it to your children!" I thought I would simply explain what's so bad about it. Then, when using the Next Generation Diet, you can probably find a place in your child's diet plan for some of the things served at your local fast food joint.

Let's look at the typical fast food hamburger. There is the bun (a simple carbohydrate), catsup (another simple carbohydrate), and then the meat itself, a small portion of protein. If you add french fries (a relatively simple carbohydrate that has been cooked in rancid, heated, partially hydrogenated vegetable oil filled with trans fatty acids), it's easy to see why the average American is eating an unhealthy diet. The emphasis in this meal is simple carbohydrates, a small amount of protein, and lots of all the wrong kinds of fats. This is not the balance the Next Generation Diet calls for.

The typical belief is that it is the fat in the meat that is the reason why your child should not be eating this fast food. The meat is the only natural substance in a fast food burger. It's all the other man-made products that surround it that, I believe, cause the problems. Think back to my new, improved version of the food pyramid. If there is an excess of simple carbohydrates and sugar in the diet, that is what will be used for energy, and the fat will be stored. If you eliminate the upper parts of the pyramid, your child's metabolism will be working so well that the fat and protein cease to be a problem. Many of my patients will have the hamburger without the bun and the catsup, or they will order the chicken and remove the skin or any breading that may be on it. There are ways of enjoying fast food in a somewhat healthy way, if you must.

how to reduce cholesterol

This same reasoning and the same pyramid explain why the cholesterol level lowers and the level of triglycerides drops precipitously. In my practice, I get this question all the time: How can cholesterol drop when a person is eating high-fat foods? Your child's body will simply burn what it is eating. There is no storage of the fat or cholesterol, so the levels drop, not increase. People can't seem to accept these simple facts because they are so brainwashed by the usual medical principle of low-fat being equated with good health and low cholesterol. At first, patients look at me incredulously when I tell them what they should be feeding their kids. But on their return visits, when I show them their child's new blood work, and they see how much weight their child has lost, I have the pleasant opportunity to see that incredulous look once again.

The truth is that your child's body will manufacture cholesterol whether you ingest it or not. It has many beneficial uses in the body. Every cell of our body needs cholesterol in order to maintain its cellular structure. Without it, our cells would fall apart and our bodies would disintegrate. In a child, this is extremely important. A child's body is growing so quickly and building new cells so rapidly, that it requires much energy and fuel. If we start depriving our children of the necessary building blocks, some of which include fat and cholesterol, then we are setting them up to not grow properly.

It's also important to realize that cholesterol is one of the body's major protective mechanisms. It is the source of one of our largest reserves of natural antioxidants. Antioxidants are substances like vitamin C and vitamin E that act as protectors of our cells and that help protect us from cancer. The liver produces cholesterol every day as a protective device. So, even if your child never ate any cholesterol, their liver would still produce it.

Only a small amount of a body's cholesterol level comes from dietary sources because only one-third of the cholesterol we eat is actually absorbed. The rest is secreted through the intestinal wall in the bowel movement. Cholesterol is only damaging to the body when it has been oxidized by exposure to heat, hence leading to free radical formation. Damaged cholesterol is found in powdered eggs and powdered milk and in meats and fats that have been burned or singed, as in grilling.

you don't want it too low

Solely from my clinical experience and intuition, I strongly believe that for many people it is unhealthy to have cholesterol levels below 150. I have treated thousands of patients, and the vast majority of those whose cholesterol was below 150 were suffering from a long-term illness, such as cancer or AIDS. Occasionally, there have been patients for whom this doesn't ring true, like long-distance runners, some athletes, and some vegetarians.

Unfortunately, things are beginning to escalate in the war against cholesterol, and I've had patients tell me that their doctor had put them on medications to lower their cholesterol level to below 150 when they presented to the doctor with a cholesterol level of 190. These medications are serious and can have potentially damaging side effects, especially to the liver, one of the most important organs in the body. Now that we, in the medical community, are becoming increasingly aware that cholesterol problems begin in childhood, how soon will it be before some company decides (with the blessings of the physician who got the glory and the funding from the study) that it is in the public's best interest for children to be on these same medications. This madness has to stop.

Pharmaceutical drugs can have potentially very harmful, even deadly side effects. Just think of fen-phen and thalidomide, to name a couple of good examples. Increasingly, I see my younger patients being placed on more and more drugs for what I see as dietary and nutritionally based disorders. In the coming chapters, I'm going to discuss some of these problems and will offer suggestions as to how to treat these very common childhood illnesses, perhaps without medication. Don't misunderstand me. Medication certainly has its place, and I couldn't practice medicine every day without them. However, you, as the consumer for your child, must know that there may be alternatives.

Admittedly, this is a somewhat controversial position. Nevertheless, I maintain that to cut fat and cholesterol from the diet completely, or nearly completely, will have potentially serious results, especially in children.

triglycerides

Many people associate triglycerides with dietary fats. The association with fats in the form of fatty acids is correct, but they are not associated with the dietary intake of fats, for the most part. Elevated triglycerides have been linked to an increased risk of coronary heart disease, and this is true. But here let me set another myth straight. Triglycerides are made in the liver from any excess sugars that have not been completely metabolized. If you think back to the discussion on insulin, you'll remember that insulin, which is the storage hormone, in its attempt to lower blood glucose, will hook together three glycogen molecules to form a triglyceride. These are the sticky kinds of fatty acids that cling to the blood vessel walls.

Think back to the Next Generation Diet food pyramid again. The source of these excess sugars is any food containing carbohydrates, but particularly refined sugar and processed carbohydrates. Triglycerides are three molecules that have been biochemically linked together. An excess level of triglycerides in the bloodstream causes a "gunking," or gluing up, of the works. Therefore, when there are too many carbohydrates in the diet, there is an excess amount of triglycerides formed and an excess amount of glue-like substances that cause the blood to thicken, hence leading to an increased risk for heart disease. These excess by-products will start to stick to places they're not supposed to, like arterial walls and cellular DNA, disrupting their function and accelerating various disease processes.

For many years it has been known that markedly high levels of triglycerides are dangerous. It is now thought to be vital to reduce the levels of triglycerides in the bloodstream even more than before. The Next Generation Diet will lower your child's triglyceride levels by reducing the amount of simple carbohydrates and sugar that they will be eating that can be converted to triglycerides by the liver.

Why not have universal cholesterol screening in children? We know high cholesterol is a diet-related problem in adults, so wouldn't it be best to start interventions as early as possible? The key to twenty-first century medicine will be prevention. And what better way to start than with our children?

If children are allowed to progress to adulthood with higher blood pressure, higher levels of LDL cholesterol (the "bad" cholesterol that is known to cause plaque formation in our arteries, hence putting us at an increased risk for cardiovascular disease), and increased risk of non-insulin-dependent diabetes mellitus due mostly to poor dietary habits, we are dooming them to a shorter life span. Children with these risk factors are absolutely associated with an increased morbidity and mortality from heart disease. And it doesn't matter if your child is the star athlete or the perennial couch potato or falls somewhere between those two. The risk is still there if these factors are present.

From my own experience as a physician, I can cite a host of examples of children whose cholesterol levels have dropped significantly while their HDLs have increased and their triglycerides have significantly decreased simply because they changed their diet. As a result, their risk of cardiovascular disease significantly diminished. This is exactly what medical science attempts to do with all their cholesterol-lowering drugs and antifat and anticholesterol campaigns, and it is something I can do far more easily and successfully, without the potentially harmful effects of drugs and the difficult-to-sustain low-fat diet. You will find this to hold true not only for overweight children, but also for your nonoverweight children.

I urge you to take advantage of the potential health benefits of the Next Generation Diet for you and your entire family.

Yeast Inflates More Than Bread

MY FIFTEEN-YEAR-OLD PATIENT KEN WAS A BOY WITH A YEAST INFECTION. I know it's hard to think of a boy having a yeast infection, but read on.

The most important part of determining what is wrong with the patient is his or her medical history. With Ken, I found that he was bothered by frequent diaper rashes as an infant, and as a toddler, he suffered from eczema. When he started going to school full time, he began experiencing frequent sinus infections, often characterized by a runny nose. The situation was always worse in the fall and in the damp weather. Because of these problems, his pediatrician regularly placed him on antibiotics for almost five months of the year. At age seven, he started to develop earaches several times during the year. Again, each time he came down with this ailment, it was treated with antibiotics. At one point the problem was so vexing that it was suggested that he have tubes placed in his ears.

Ken was always a well-behaved child, but his father did describe him as being somewhat on the cranky side. He had regularly performed well in school up to the past year when he started to wheeze and experience shortness of breath, both symptoms of asthma. At the same time, his concentration started to decline, and he became perpetually tired. Out of desperation, after having been to see several other doctors, each of whom handed out one prescription or another for various medications, his parents brought him to see me. By the time Ken arrived at my office, he was taking six different medications, none of which seemed to be doing any good. Needless to say, his parents were at their wits' end.

As I listened to his story, it soon became clear to me what was at the root of Ken's problem, so much so that I almost did not need to do any confirmatory blood tests. However, I did perform the tests anyway, in large part so that I would have proof for his parents. The candida antibody test, along with a cytotoxic food sensitivity test, confirmed my suspicions of a candida (yeast) infection. The candida antibody test shows if your child has built up any antibodies to the candida, which is a sign of whether your child has ever been exposed to it. The test measures three different antibodies so a doctor is able to tell if your child had an infection or has an active infection.

When I gave them the results, his parents were relieved that I had been able to find a reason for their son's change in behavior; yet, they had no idea what I was talking about. I then explained to them what yeast is, how Ken could have gotten it, and, more importantly, what we needed to do to get rid of it and do away with their son's symptoms.

Ken's case was an extreme and dramatic example, in that he exhibited so many symptoms. I can relate many other cases that have some but not all of these symptoms. The fact is, your child does not have to exhibit all the symptoms I've just described in order to have problems with yeast. I use two symptoms or more as a general guideline. If the child exhibits two or more of the symptoms I've just described, I would feel justified in placing them on a yeast-free diet.

Within two weeks after I placed Ken on Phase 1 of the Next Generation Diet (because he was twenty pounds overweight) with a yeast restriction, many of his symptoms had disappeared, and those that were left had begun to slowly dissipate. Immediately, I was able to eliminate three of his asthma drugs, and within six months, Ken was on absolutely no medications at all. Most importantly, he was feeling better than ever. Because Ken no longer had a weight problem by this time, I moved him to Phase 3 of the diet and slowly began to remove his yeast restrictions. I also prescribed a series of nutritional supplements that aid in the elimination of candida.

what is yeast?

Candida albicans is a naturally occurring yeast that lives in the mucous membranes of the gastrointestinal and the genitourinary tracts, as well as on the skin. The gastrointestinal tract is one of the largest components of the human body and is comprised of the mouth, the rectum, and everything in between: the esophagus, stomach, and small and large intestines. The genitourinary tract includes the kidneys, ureters, and urethras. Candida only becomes a problem when it is allowed to overgrow and take up more space than it should.

Candida albicans is an opportunistic mold and yeast fungus. It is considered opportunistic because it will only cause a problem when the body's defense mechanisms are impaired. If this happens, the candida can then overgrow, causing the problems I've previously described. Also, because it lacks chlorophyll, it is not able to produce its own food and acts like a parasite in our bodies.

Antibiotics, birth control pills, steroids (such as prednisone), pregnancy, and diabetes can encourage the overgrowth of yeast in the body. As far as our children are concerned, so long as they are healthy, the major reason that would cause the yeast, or the candida, to overgrow is their diet. The average diet of a child contains too much sugar and simple refined carbohydrates. The refined carbohydrates (which as you'll recall are metabolized as sugar), along with the sugar itself, will feed the yeast and lead to an overgrowth. The sugar is its source of fuel. Think of a forest fire that can't stop because there's just so much fuel to feed it. The parents of my young patients often wonder, "Where could my kids possibly have picked up such a thing?" The answer I give often startles them: "You need look no further than your own medicine cabinet and your own refrigerator."

I honestly believe yeast, or more precisely, candida albicans, can be extremely detrimental to the health of many people, including children. In my practice, I have seen this affect my patients in many ways, including the inability to lose weight. In fact, it can be a prime culprit in this regard, so much so, that if your child does not lose weight after being on the diet outlined in the previous chapters, I would suggest that you try to eliminate all foods that contain yeast, the foods that can help promote an overgrowth of the candida.

The reason I've dedicated an entire chapter to this problem is because of all the health implications. Recurrent ear infections, behavioral and learning problems, asthma, and allergies are all on the rise and have reached epidemic proportions. In my clinical experience, I feel these may be related to a yeast problem that is one of the causes, for the most part, clinically overlooked by most physicians.

There are many symptoms that can indicate a yeast infection, or more specifically, a yeast overgrowth. Some of the gastrointestinal complaints include bowel problems, such as bloating, gas or flatulence, indigestion, or heartburn. Many younger children often complain of not feeling well after they eat.

A typical complaint that I'm sure you've run into is, "Mommy, my tummy hurts." Children, especially the younger ones, often cannot put into words some of the things they are feeling as well as adults can. Consequently, as a parent, you have to be able to look beyond the words. If this happens often to your child and you can come up with no other logical explanation, then I would consider yeast as a possible cause for this complaint.

The next set of symptoms that may be attributable to yeast are the classic allergy reactions, including asthma, hives, runny nose, sinus problems, acne, eczema, and earaches. Yeast may not be the direct cause of *all* the cases of these illnesses, but it should at least be considered and treated in any child suffering from any of these conditions.

Unfortunately, conventional medicine has determined that candida plays no role in causing these illnesses, hence money goes into finding new drugs to treat the symptoms, not to discovering potential underlying causes.

the problem with antibiotics

Antibiotics play a role in modern medicine, but it is the overprescription of these wonder drugs that has me concerned. Many physicians can readily attest to this fact. Only recently are some doctors willing to at least admit that this kind of overprescription occurs. Now we need to find out if it causes any harm. Personally, I find it hard to believe that it doesn't. Think about it. Those drugs are meant to kill things. As a result, it only stands to reason that they must have a powerful effect on our bodies. The antibiotics not only kill pathogenic (disease-causing) bacteria, they also kill beneficial bacteria, our bodies' own natural flora, the combination of several different species of bacteria that live in the gastrointestinal tract to help in the digestion of food and the absorption of nutrients.

Candida normally lives side-by-side with all the other microorganisms in the gastrointestinal tract. But when the good bacteria in your intestines are destroyed when your child takes antibiotics, this intestinal equilibrium is upset. The candida (a fungus, which is not killed by antibiotics) now has room to multiply and to take over your child's digestive tract.

Most women reading this book are probably nodding to themselves now because they know that when they take antibiotics, the antibiotics will destroy the good bacteria in the vagina, and they stand a very good chance of contracting a vaginal yeast infection. This same thing will occur in your child's digestive tract every time he or she takes antibiotics.

Although there hasn't been an overwhelming amount of study conducted in this area, there has been some scientific literature that has examined this phenomenon. In a study in the *Journal of Allergy and Clinical Immunology*, published in January 1994, researchers from the University of Virginia found that oral antifungal medication, such as ketoconazole and fluconazole, provided help to a number of patients suffering from intrinsic asthma. It would stand to reason that there may be a fungal component to this illness because those two drugs kill candida and all other forms of yeast. Other studies have reported favorable responses to diseases such as psoriasis, autism, and chronic depression by using antifungal medication.

As you can probably tell from the symptoms I've pointed out, yeast is not just an issue for the overweight child. It is an important health consideration for every child.

Some of the most common symptoms in the younger group include crankiness, constant colds, excessive diaper rash, sleep problems, ear infections, problems with their attention span, and hyperactivity. The most common symptoms in this younger age group by far are ear infections and colic. Unfortunately, these earaches are routinely treated with antibiotics by conventional doctors, which in fact further exacerbates the situation, setting the stage for even more candida proliferation and overgrowth.

Older children and teenagers will report irritability, fatigue, a "spaced out" feeling, poor school performance, headaches, and even depression.

controlling yeast without drugs

The most therapeutic program for treating candida overgrowth is an adjusted diet, accompanied by nutritional supplements, such as probiotics (good bacteria that promote health) and antifungal elements that will greatly enhance the effectiveness of the diet.

The object of this process is to ultimately restore the body's balance of bacterial flora. The best way of doing this is to eliminate all sugars from your child's diet. This should be relatively easy for those of you who have read this far because you know how to do just that. Now you must learn not only to eliminate sugar from the diet, but all yeast as well.

Identifying food products that contain yeast is fairly easy. Just remember, everything that rises contains yeast. This includes all breads except those that specifically state that they are yeast-free.

In this war against yeast, you will also need to eliminate high-carbohydrate vegetables like potatoes, sweet potatoes, peas, corn, and lima beans. Another category of food that must be avoided for children on a yeast-free diet is fruit of any kind. This includes fruit juices. Remember, sugar is still sugar, no matter what form it takes.

One other food product that must be avoided is cheese of any kind, but especially the aged cheeses. Cheeses have undergone a process of fermentation. Some cheeses, like blue cheese and Roquefort, even contain molds themselves. The soft cheeses like cream cheese, cottage cheese, pot cheese, farmer cheese, and ricotta, do not contain yeast, but they do contain a small amount of sugar. It is for this reason that they should be avoided.

Mushrooms, because they are a type of fungus, must also be avoided, as should fermented food of any kind. This includes vinegar, soy sauce, sauerkraut, sour cream, mayonnaise, and mustard. The last two must be dropped from your diet because they contain vinegar and may contain sugars. If you have any doubts, just check the label of the food in question.

❖ Foods to Be Avoided on a Yeast-Free Diet ❖

Alcoholic beverages

All foods that contain sugar

Barbecue sauce

Biscuits

Breads

Buttermilk

Candy

Catsup

Cereals with sugar

Cheese

Cookies

Cottage cheese

Crackers

Dried and cured foods

Dried fruits

Dried roasted nuts

Fermented beverages

Flour

Frozen or canned citrus fruit and juices

Hamburger and hot dog buns

Horseradish

Mayonnaise

Milk

Mushrooms

Olives

Pastries

Pickles

Pretzels

Root beer

Rolls

Sauerkraut

Smoked foods

Sour cream

Soy sauce

Store-bought salad dressings

Teas

Tomato sauce

Truffles

Vinegar

Note: Milk is not allowed on a yeast-free diet because of the sugar in the milk. This is the same reason that I don't like to add yogurt to the very strict early stage of the yeast-free diet.

A yeast-free diet is something that needs to be continued for at least three months, that is only if your child has strictly adhered to the diet, without cheating even once. Because this is such a difficult restriction for most patients, I generally recommend your child stay on a yeast-free diet for six months. It takes a long time to cure this sensitivity to the yeast, although your child should feel significantly better within the first month. The longer your child can handle the restrictions, the better it is to keep them on it.

After that period of time has elapsed, a transition period should take place. This will serve to not overwhelm your child's system with foods that contain yeast or sugar products. I start with the resumption of fruit such as berries, melons, and grapefruit (one-half cup serving for three days per week). After two weeks, I would allow fresh cheeses, like cottage, ricotta, farmer, pot, or cream cheese (a 2-ounce serving four days per week for two weeks). If after this first month, none of the original

❖ Foods That Can Be Eaten on a Yeast-Free Diet ❖

Now that we know all the things your child can't eat, here are some of
the foods that are permitted.

WHOLE GRAINS	BREADS	CEREALS	WHOLE GRAIN PASTAS
Rice—short, medium, and long grain (brown preferable, but white may be used)	Yeast-free breads like sourdough, rye, essene, spelt, kamut, and multigrain	Hot wheat	Whole wheat pasta (also called Udon)
		Oat	
		Rice	Artichoke pasta
		Mixed-grain cereals	Corn pasta (wheat-free)
	Corn tortillas	Cold cereals: shredded wheat, puffed wheat, puffed millet, puffed corn, puffed rice, puffed kashi	Rice pasta (wheat-free)
Cracked wheat	Chapatis (made from wheat)		
Bulgar wheat			Buckwheat pasta (also called Soba)
Couscous			
Millet			
Oats			
Barley			
Buckwheat groats (kasha)			
Quinoa			
Amaranth			

symptoms reappear, I would then gradually allow regular aged cheeses
and then lastly breads that contain yeast. The more slowly you reintroduce these products back into your child's diet, the more lasting and
successful the outcome will be. Remember, your child has now gone
without these foods for several months. Chances are the desire for these
foods has also abated. There is no rush. After all, we are trying to
achieve a lifetime of success.

other ways to control yeast in your child

Diet, of course, is the most important aspect in the control of yeast. There are, however, other things you can do that will aid your child in the fight against yeast. There are many natural products that enhance yeast elimination. And, if I feel yeast is a problem for any of my patients, I'll often add several of these products to my patient's nutritional supplement program. Later in this book, I'll share some of the more common nutritional supplements I prescribe for my patients.

Normally, I would advise you to see your pediatrician if you felt yeast was an issue with your child, but, as I've said before, few physicians are convinced yeast is of concern. Consequently, your pediatrician, unless he or she is exceptionally broadminded, would probably tell you not to worry about yeast. But you should.

I will list several natural products you may want to try, if you feel this is a possibility. However, I would feel more comfortable if you tried to find a physician in your area who is familiar with complementary medicine. I practice complementary medicine. I use the best of all possible worlds—conventional and alternative medical techniques—in order to heal the patient. They are not two separate entities. One is meant to complement the other.

Supplements

Basically, there are three ways of attacking this problem. The first is through supplements that will destroy the yeast cell itself. The ones I use for my pediatric patients are garlic and caprylic acid. Garlic is thought to inhibit candida by damaging the structure and integrity of the yeast cell wall. This will cause the yeast cell to rupture and die. Allicin, one of garlic's key ingredients, is believed to provide many of garlic's antimicrobial properties. For children weighing under 100 pounds, I generally use 100 milligrams per day. For every 20 pounds heavier your child is, I would increase the dose by 50 milligrams. You must give your child the kind of garlic that has an odor. It is the allicin, which is the active ingredient in the garlic, that produces this odor. In the smaller doses used in children, the odor is mild, and so it usually will not make your child's breath smell.

Caprylic acid is a fatty acid that has been shown to have antifungal and antimicrobial properties. It is a medium-chain fatty acid commonly used to fight microorganism overgrowth. It is naturally produced in the body in very small amounts, and therapeutic (i.e., larger) doses must be given by mouth in the form of supplementation. This fatty acid is also found in butter and in coconut and palm oils. Because it is naturally produced by the body, I have no problem giving this to my patients as young as eight years old. The dose I use is calculated according to the weight of the child. It is approximately 100 milligrams once per day if your child is under 75 pounds; 100 milligrams twice per day if your child is 75 to 100 pounds; and 100 milligrams three times per day if your child is above 100 pounds.

Again, a note of caution when it comes to giving your child any kind of supplements: remember, these are general guidelines for you to use at home. I always recommend that you use supplements as you would use any other medication, under the advice of a physician. There can be side effects, and I certainly would not want anyone to suffer because of something they may have read in this book. As you probably know by now, my ultimate goal is for everyone to be healthy. Help me achieve this goal by not using any supplements that I've recommended in this book unwisely. All my patients at the Atkins Center are treated as individuals, and the dosages of any medication or supplements that I prescribe are adjusted for these variables. So, please be careful when administering either medications or supplements at home, without the advice of a physician. And, if your child experiences any unpleasant side effects, consult a physician immediately.

how to use probiotics

The second way of attacking any yeast problem is to replenish the bowel tract with the normal bacteria, thereby restoring your child's body to its original balance. Probiotics are essentially the opposite of antibiotics. These are the good, healthy, useful bacteria that unfortunately get removed along with the harmful bacteria whenever your child takes an antibiotic. It is necessary for the human intestine to maintain a critical balance among all the different bacteria present in the digestive system. Whenever one becomes unbalanced, symptoms may occur. After all, these bacteria play a vital role in supporting and protecting intestinal and immune function.

The three most common protective strains of bacteria are Lactobacillus acidophilus, Bifidobacterium bifidum, and Lactobacillus bulgaricus. Generally, I prescribe a product that contains all three.

In my younger patients, I will use a weight-related dose. For children under 100 pounds, I will use 1 million units of each probiotic, divided over each meal. For every additional 25 pounds your child may weigh, I add 500,000 units of each to a maximum of 6 million units per day in divided doses. These may seem like small doses to physicians familiar with the use of nutritional supplements like these; however, I will always err on the side of caution. Because you will be doing this on your own, without any input other than what you're now reading, please adhere to the lower doses.

Top Five Tips for Controlling Yeast

1. Avoid antibiotics.
2. If your child requires antibiotics, make sure to replace the beneficial bacteria by using probiotics, such as acidophilus and bifidus, during the entire time your child is on the antibiotic and then for ten days, after the antibiotic course has been completed.
3. Follow a yeast-free diet.
4. Avoid sugar.
5. Avoid processed foods.

drugs

Some physicians feel that these yeast infections should be treated with conventional medications. There are several antifungal medications currently available and being used. The safest one for children, I feel, is Nystatin. I generally do not treat this way, but if asked to recommend treatment, I would advise 250,000 units by mouth each time your child is given an antibiotic. Once the antibiotic is finished, I would continue to give the Nystatin for two weeks. This helps discourage the growth of candida, while allowing the probiotics to work. The probiotics, as I mentioned earlier, must be taken any time your child is given antibiotics.

The other commonly prescribed drugs for controlling yeast are fluconazole and ketoconazole. However, I save these drugs for my adult patients. There have been some negative side effects with respect to the liver associated with these drugs, and I feel they are only indicated for very serious cases. I have never used these drugs in children, and probably never will.

acne: facing the problem

Peter, fifteen years old, visited me because he had a bad case of acne. His pediatrician had placed him on antibiotics for almost a year and had tried all the facial creams on the market. Still his condition only got worse. His weight was normal, but when I questioned him about his eating habits, I found that his diet was loaded with soda, fruit juice, and all kinds of candy, along with a huge amount of processed foods, the typical teenage male diet.

The solution to his problem was a bit more complicated because I could tell, just from reviewing his history, that he almost certainly had a systemic yeast infection, not only from the number of antibiotics that he had taken over the past year, but also because of the outrageous amounts of sugar and refined carbohydrates he was ingesting.

I explained the Phase 2 diet to him, and he just looked at me in a way that any parent of a fifteen-year-old boy can immediately relate to. "There's no way I can do that," he exclaimed.

I looked back at him the way a thirty-five-year-old can and replied, "If you want your face to clear up in time for the prom three months from now, you have no choice." I made him a promise: "Peter, if your face isn't at least 75 percent better than it is now, you can take my car for a spin."

Now, I was in trouble, because there was no way I was going to let a fifteen-year-old boy drive my car. But, as it turned out—as I knew it would—I didn't have to. His skin did clear up, and he wound up taking the most popular girl in school to the prom. Three months prior to his visit to me, he would not have even been able to consider talking to this "beauty," as he described her, let alone have the courage to ask her out on a date.

As a result of the change in his diet, not only did Peter's complexion improve, but so did his self-esteem, which is no small accomplishment. In fact, there is nothing more rewarding to me than to see how the loss of weight or the attainment of a healthier state positively affects the lives of my patients.

After a period of adjustment, kids learn to love their new nutritional guidelines and how their lives have changed for the good. As a result, they almost never go off the diet, which is something I wish I could say for my adult patients, who are always finding one excuse or another to cheat.

The supplement program I designed for Peter included the anticandida supplements like mycocidin, caprylic acid, and grapefruit seed extract. I also placed him on the probiotics, a combination of acidophilus, lactobacillus, and bifidus. His program included essential fatty acids, such as flaxseed oil, GLA, and fish oils. I then added vitamin C, beta-carotene, vitamin A, and garlic.

This may sound like a lot, but Peter's case was very severe and it did work. When the initial problem starts to subside, I will decrease the number of supplements slowly over a course of time, until the problem is completely resolved. I deliberately avoid mentioning doses because I don't want you to use this book as a self-treatment guide when it comes to supplements. If you would like to help your child with these supplements, you should consult a physician who is knowledgeable about the use of these nutrients.

Acne Treatment in Short

- ❖ Phase 1 or Phase 2 diet, as appropriate
- ❖ Elimination of any food sensitivities
- ❖ Yeast restriction
- ❖ Nutritional supplements that include beta-carotene, garlic, caprylic acid, omega-3 fatty acids, and others

Just because your child may be experiencing some of the symptoms of a candida overgrowth does not mean he or she has it. If you are not sure, restrict yeast for seven to ten days. If your child's symptoms get better, then I would stay on the yeast-free diet; if not, another problem may be plaguing your child.

But no matter what you read here, please remember and act on this caveat: *if your child is not well, please bring him or her to the attention of a qualified physician.* The treatment plan for each child—especially if he or she is not feeling well—must be individualized and as such requires a face-to-face visit with a qualified physician. If you fail to do this, you are running the risk of complications that might arise from not getting the proper medical care your child.

Allergies and
Food Sensitivities

PATRICK WAS AN ELEVEN-YEAR-OLD BOY WHO WAS BROUGHT TO MY OFFICE by his parents who were concerned about his allergies, the symptoms of which seemed to consist primarily of a runny nose, stuffy head, occasional itchy eyes, and a scratchy throat. These were not seasonal problems that occurred in the spring and summer when most kids get allergy symptoms. Patrick had these symptoms all the time.

His parents were tired of giving Patrick nasal decongestants and antihistamines, which never seemed to work, and often made him more irritable, sleepy, or hyperexcited. By the time they came to me, they were frustrated that no doctor was getting to the cause of the problem.

After a thorough history and physical examination, I performed several blood tests on Patrick. These consisted of routine chemistries and a hematology test that any physician would order; but in addition, I ordered a glucose tolerance test, a candida antibody test, and a cyto-toxic food sensitivity test. All his tests turned out normal, except for a mild reaction to the candida antibody and several food sensitivities to corn, wheat, rye, oats, and broccoli.

I suggested to Patrick's parents that food sensitivities could well be the cause of many of their son's symptoms. I outlined a diet for him that eliminated all the foods to which he was sensitive. I did not place him on a yeast-restricted diet similar to the one outlined in the previous chapter because his candida antibody levels were not high enough to justify that restriction. Patrick was not overweight, so I placed him on the Phase 2 diet.

In addition to the diet, I also placed him on several nutritional sup-plements that may act as natural antihistamines, such as quercetin, vit-amin C, vitamin A, garlic and the omega-3 fatty acids.

By the end of the first week of the elimination of these foods from his diet, Patrick's head and nasal passages began to clear. He had never felt better, and his parents were extremely grateful.

the food sensitivity–yeast bridge

There is often an association between candida or yeast infection and the development of food sensitivities. At this time, I'd like to take just a moment to explain the proposed mechanism behind the develop-ment of food sensitivities.

Candida albicans really has two life forms: the yeast and the fungus. The yeast state is essentially noninvasive. The fungus, on the other hand, produces rootlike structures called rhizoids, which can penetrate the intestinal lining. Think back to a biology class experiment that per-mitted mold to grow on bread or to a time when you've left unrefrig-erated bread in the cabinet for too long. Those greenish, hairlike growths are the rhizomes, or rhizoids.

When these rhizomes penetrate the lining of your intestines, the closed system is disrupted which allows undigested dietary proteins to move into the bloodstream. If this happens to your child, his or her immune system will perceive these undigested proteins as foreign, something is where it should not be. The warning bell sounds, and your child's immune system will create an antibody against this substance so it can be eliminated. Once this antibody has been produced, your body will elicit a similar response each time you come into contact with that substance. This means that your body will try to destroy this foreign invader each time. This has been described as "leaky-gut" syndrome, most notably by Leo Galland, M.D. This same syndrome is now being recognized by many leading gastroenterologists across the country, and more research is currently being done on this fascinating topic.

The reaction that takes place in your child's body is similar to the reaction that occurs in your child's immune system when he or she suffers from a cold or has been inoculated against a disease.

is a food sensitivity really an allergy?

There is a difference between a food sensitivity and a true food allergy. Many parents reading this book who have a child who is truly allergic to a particular food know how terrifying the experience can be the first time you realize your child is having an allergic reaction. This reaction can be experienced as anything from rashes, asthma, and hives to something more life-threatening like an inability to breathe (anaphylaxis).

To test for true food allergies, your child's pediatrician or allergist would do a series of skin tests, using a prick or puncture method to determine your child's level of reactivity to certain food products. This can also be done for environmental allergies such as ragweed, dust mites, and other common allergens.

North American children are most commonly allergic to milk, eggs, peanuts, and wheat. Scientists believe that many of these food allergies eventually will be outgrown. However, the peanut allergy tends to be the most long-lasting allergy and will almost always last a lifetime. Other foods that are closely associated with lifelong food allergies include tree nuts, like almonds, brazil, cashews, filberts, pecans, pistachios, and walnuts; fish; shellfish, especially crab, crayfish, prawns, shrimp, and lobster; and seeds, such as sesame and caraway. Should a true allergy exist, these foods must be strictly avoided.

what is a food sensitivity?

A food sensitivity exists when the body responds in a negative way to an ostensible intruder, even though the person may not have an allergy per se to that intruder. Many parents think their child does not suffer from food sensitivities because they have never noticed a reaction to a particular food. A test for food sensitivities does not look for outright allergies. If your child is allergic to a particular food, you are generally aware of the symptoms, like wheezing, hives, or itchiness. Food sensitivities are far more subtle and more often than not you will never notice a direct correlation until that particular food is removed from your child's diet.

In my clinical experience, food sensitivities may be related to many of the most common childhood health disorders, such as asthma, seasonal allergies, and learning and behavioral problems, among other things. Because the correlation is so subtle, it is often overlooked by most doctors. In fact, most conventional (allopathic) physicians do not even believe in the validity of food-sensitivity testing and, therefore, may not be able to adequately evaluate your child.

In my pediatric population, I have found the most common food sensitivity to be to grains, such as corn, wheat, oats, rye, and barley. These grains all contain gluten, and these are probably a big part of your child's current diet. I recommend that many of my young patients eliminate these substances from their diet if they are experiencing any allergy-type symptoms to see if those symptoms can be easily eliminated.

could this be a cold or an infection?

Of course, some symptoms may represent a cold or an infection, but, remember, a cold or an infection is not something that will last more than a few days or a week. A cold or an infection is not something that should recur on an almost daily basis. The average child is expected to get between seven and ten colds during the cold and flu season. From my experience, I wonder how many of these are really colds or the flu or just an exacerbation of their allergy symptoms.

An important thing to keep in mind is that not every runny nose or nagging cough is necessarily an infection. More likely, this is indicative of an allergy or a sensitivity. Approximately 30 percent of children who present with recurrent respiratory symptoms are having allergy attacks. Another large percentage of these children will have a viral cause of their symptoms. And remember, viruses are not killed by antibiotics. These children often do not have a fever and will not respond to antibiotics.

Physicians also often prescribe the newest antibiotic, which is generally a very broad-spectrum product. These change very frequently, but the latest prescribing fad is for drugs like azithromycin or clarithromycin. Medications like these will kill anything in their path. It's like using a shotgun to kill a fly. Instead, it's far safer and more efficient for physicians to go back to using the older, more narrow-spectrum antibiotics, such as penicillin or erythromycin if they need to be used at all.

Allergy Treatment in Short

- Phase 1 diet, if your child is overweight
- Phase 2 diet, if your child is not overweight
- Nutritional supplements, such as quercetin, garlic, vitamins A and C, and manganese, to name a few
- Yeast restriction where appropriate
- Food sensitivity testing
- If such tests are unavailable, then all wheat, corn, rye, oat, barley, and sugar must be eliminated from the diet.

For the most part an allergy or a food sensitivity can be treated in the same way: eliminating the allergen from the environment or the diet. It seems relatively easy, yet because food sensitivities are so subtle, they can easily go undetected for many years, even into adulthood. As someone who practices nutritional medicine, I have found the testing for food sensitivities, and their elimination, to be an invaluable tool in the road to good health for many of my patients. My advice is to keep all this in mind when your child has some minor symptoms that never seem to go away.

Asthma

S<small>ARA WAS AN ELEVEN-YEAR-OLD GIRL</small> who was having an increasingly difficult time controlling her asthma. It was an allergic asthma, and so it was always worse in the spring and the fall, or whenever she came into contact with a new environment. Sara was only about five pounds overweight, so obesity was not an issue. Her parents brought her to the office because they wanted her to be off the steroid medication that her pediatrician had claimed was necessary for Sara to be able to breathe properly. Understandably, her parents were quite concerned with the possible long-term side effects that have been associated with steroid use, such as weight gain and diabetes.

After taking a thorough history and giving her a physical examination, I performed a series of blood tests on her. These tests included the candida antibody assays and a cytotoxic food sensitivity test. Sara scored very highly on the antibody assay test and also demonstrated food sensitivities to candida, molds, wheat, rye, oat, barley, and buckwheat. This did not surprise me because it is a typical pattern of children with asthma and allergies. The thing that did surprise me, however, was how high she scored on these tests. Usually, when a child is on steroids, his or her immune system is suppressed, and he or she can't mount a good response to the test. As a result, I am usually left with a false negative reading. This was not the case with Sara, so I knew she probably had very strong food sensitivities and would likely be helped by my diet.

I placed Sara on a yeast-free version of the Phase 2 diet and gave her the good bacteria (i.e., the probiotics) to take with each meal, along with garlic, caprylic acid, vitamin C, and other antioxidants. Within two weeks, Sara no longer had need of her inhalers, and three months later, we were able to remove all of her medications. There are still times when Sara needs to use her inhalers: usually, when she is in a new or moldy environment, is exposed to a new pet, or even occasionally out of the blue. However, she uses them now only intermittently, and her pulmonary function tests could not be better.

Don't be fooled into thinking that the process with Sara was as smooth as it might sound. There were setbacks and times where we had to raise the amount of medications she took. However, eventually she was able to come off all the medications, and as of today, one and a half years later, she has not had any medical problems deriving from her asthma.

has asthma come from out of the blue?

In the past few decades, asthma, once an obscure allergic syndrome, has emerged as one of the nation's leading health concerns. It now affects 5 million children, and the number of sufferers has increased by 61 percent since the early 1980s. Young grade school children often go to school armed with inhalers and medications the same way I used to go to school armed with the latest baseball cards. They can probably also tell you their airflow rate in liters per minute (a common measure of how well they're breathing) as accurately as their telephone numbers.

Despite years of research, scientists have yet to determine the primary cause for asthma, and, truth be known, if you asked ten different doctors, you'd probably get at least that many answers as to its origin. What we do know is that asthma is the constriction of the small air vessels (bronchioles) in your child's lungs, causing him or her to make a wheezing noise and to have difficulty breathing. This reaction occurs when an irritant sets off a histamine reaction causing these bronchioles to constrict, making it difficult to move air in and out of the lungs.

Interestingly enough, asthma is not usually a problem in nonindustrialized societies. For instance, a 1991 study of children in Zimbabwe showed that only 1 in 1,000 children living in a rural area suffered from asthma, whereas 1 in 17 children living in the capital city of Harare suffered from asthma symptoms.

The easy answer is to attribute this to air pollution, which is obviously present in a larger degree in an urban area. However, the air in our major cities is notably cleaner now than it has been in several decades, and yet there has been a marked increase in the number of cases of asthma.

The next place to look is at the quality of indoor air. Most Americans spend most of their time indoors, with children in this country averaging a mere two hours of outdoor activity daily. The majority of the rest of the time is spent inside, gazing interactively at the screens of personal computers and televisions. Homes have become more tightly sealed due to energy concerns, and this decreases the amount of fresh air that enters a home each hour. Outside air is known to be more harmful when it is stagnant than when it is circulating, and the same is true of indoor air. Because there are so many common household hazards, from cleaning supplies to dry cleaning residue, and because homes are so tightly sealed, once innocuous contaminants can now build to such high levels in the stagnant indoor air that they become a source of harm.

I believe that another possible key to understanding the increase in the cases of asthma can, once again, be traced to the rise in the use of antibiotics that our children have been given. While these antibiotics may well kill harmful bacteria, they may also act to weaken the body's immune system. Since I was a child, the incidence of asthma has risen dramatically. What has also risen since I was a child is the use of antibiotics for every childhood complaint. Coincidence? Perhaps. But I truly believe that this connection can be made.

In addition to the rise in the use of antibiotics, another mostly overlooked possible concern in regard to asthma is the effect of food sensitivities. Because asthma has an allergic component and food sensitivities may cause an allergy-type reaction, there is a possibility that we are seeing more cases of asthma simply as a result of our children's immune system being bombarded on a daily basis by these allergens. This potential decrease in the effectiveness of your child's immune system may be one of the many causes of the more than 60 percent increase in the incidence of asthma since the early 1980s.

For my asthmatic patients, I recommend several things. The first step is to put them on a yeast-free diet to immediately eliminate one potential cause for an asthmatic attack. If the child is overweight, he is placed on the Phase 1 diet, and if not, Phase 2. The second step is to conduct a cytotoxic food sensitivity test that will help me determine the foods to which my patient may be sensitive. The third step is to prescribe a series of the following nutritional supplements that I've seen work many times and for which there is some scientific confirmation.

The *Archives of Pediatrics and Adolescent Medicine* found that a single (large) dose of vitamin C (2,000 mg) before exercise prevented exercise-induced asthma. Because 70 percent of asthmatic children have this type of asthma and 98 percent of children attending an asthma clinic complained of symptoms during exercise, this certainly seems like something that should be given to all asthmatic kids.

Because other antioxidants have been shown to decrease a person's susceptibility to the effects of air pollution, I also recommend the following antioxidant supplements for children with asthma: Vitamin C – 2 to 4 grams daily, depending on the age and weight of your child. The less your child weighs, the lower the dose. However, as a general rule, start your child with 250 milligrams (0.25 grams) of vitamin C and increase this by 250 milligrams every other day until you've reached 4,000 milligrams (4 grams). If your child develops diarrhea from the vitamin C, then you know they can't tolerate any more than what you're already giving them.

I also prescribe 400 IU of vitamin E and 25,000 IU of beta-carotene in the natural carotenoid form (this form will have all the carotenoids in the mixture and is believed to be a more beneficial product than Beta carotene alone). Also, because most of my patients with asthma have been found to have a problem with yeast, I usually prescribe the supplements I described in Chapter 21.

You will find that some herbal practitioners would advocate the use of ephedra for the treatment of asthma. Ephedra is biochemically similar to common asthma medications, such as aminophylline, and it has been used successfully for many years in Chinese medicine. However, because I find it difficult to determine the proper dosage in children, it is not something I can recommend. If I wanted to use a substance like that, I would use it in a medication form, such as theophylline.

Because most asthmatics have an allergenic component to their disease, it seems logical to discuss the connection between asthma, yeast, and food sensitivities. In my clinical experience, I have found this to be true. What works for my patients is the elimination of many foods or substances to which I've found my patients to be sensitive, such as all grains that contain gluten (wheat, rye, oat, barley, and corn,) sugar, and all yeast-containing products.

Foods are not the only things to which children may be sensitive. There are a whole range of other things, including dust mites, molds and animal dander. Consequently, it may be necessary, even desirable, to have your child tested for these things. (For this you will need to seek the advice of an allergist.)

Beyond elimination of any and all potential allergens, there are also many nutritional supplements you can give your child to improve their allergy-related problems. In addition to the ones I've already mentioned, I use vitamin A, in a dose of 10,000 to 30,000 IU per day (although beta-carotene is the precursor of vitamin A, they work differently in the body, and I have often found it necessary to use both in my asthmatic population); quercetin, or the other citrus bioflavonoids, in a dose of 40 milligrams three times per day (quercetin, catechin, rutin, and hesperidin are thought to possess antihistaminic properties); pantethine, in a dose of 125 to 1,000 milligrams per day (it is thought to act as an antiallergen). The smaller doses should be used for the smaller child. Remember, always start with the smallest dose I recommend and build up slowly until you see the maximum improvement.

Asthma Treatment in Short

- ❖ Phase 1 diet, yeast-free, for overweight children
- ❖ Phase 2 diet, yeast-free, for nonoverweight children
- ❖ Food sensitivity testing
- ❖ If such tests are unavailable, then all wheat, corn, rye, oat, barley, and sugar must be eliminated from the diet.
- ❖ Nutritional supplements in the doses described above, including vitamin C, vitamin A, beta-carotene, quercetin, and vitamin E

success

With this combination—diet, antiyeast supplements, antioxidants, and the nutritional supplements I've just mentioned—I've achieved a pretty significant success rate without having to resort to drugs such as steroids or antihistamines that have no right being in a child's school bag.

Many children have come to my office with complaints of asthma. Most of them are using several inhalers and taking oral medications to cope with the symptoms of their disease. But within a few weeks—sometimes a few months—of being on my diet, along with the nutritional supplements that I feel are necessary, the vast majority of them are totally free of some if not all of these medications. This is a feeling of great accomplishment for me, and I hope some of you will have the same success. Just keep in mind that it is not as easy as it may appear, and often I've spent months of adjusting foods and supplements in order to achieve my success stories.

eczema

Eczema is a mild red rash that generally appears on the skin but may develop into deeper red patches that are itchy. They may even get infected and start to ooze if your child scratches them too hard. Infantile eczema is generally associated with childhood asthma, and that's why I'm mentioning it in this chapter. Most children I see suffering with asthma will have had eczema as an infant or a very young child.

Again, although quite difficult to treat, I've had clinical success with placing children suffering from eczema on a yeast-free, Phase 1 or Phase 2 diet (depending on weight), while using the nutritional supplements I've previously described for a yeast problem. In addition, I would add omega-3 and omega-6 fatty acids to the diet of children with eczema. This can be taken in the form of GLA capsules, borage oil capsules, fish oil capsules, and flaxseed oil capsules. I usually recommend one to six of these per day, spread evenly throughout the day. The strength is 250 to 1,000 milligrams, depending on the size of the child: the general rule is the smaller (not necessarily younger) child gets lower doses.

The Common Cold, Earaches, and Other Complaints

Nine-year-old Paula was brought to my office because of the frequency of her colds. It seemed to her parents that she was sick every other week, sometimes for months at a time. Because of this, her pediatrician placed her on antibiotics at least twice per month, meaning there was probably ten days out of the month when she wasn't on antibiotics. These antibiotics did nothing for her because she continued to suffer from these colds.

In Paula's blood tests, the only interesting thing to report was her lack of candida antibodies. With the amount of antibiotics she was taking, I would have thought the opposite. Paula was overweight, so she went on the Phase 1 diet, and two weeks after I prescribed a course of nutritional supplementation, virtually all of Paula's cold symptoms were gone.

the common cold

Before I explain my course of treatment with Paula, let's talk about the common cold, which most children, especially the younger ones, suffer from several times a year.

The incidence of the common cold in our children is on the rise. One possible reason is our increasing reliance on day care. This puts children in close contact with each other, thus allowing for germs to spread very easily from one to the other. As many as six to ten minor, often viral respiratory infections per year are not uncommon, nor is a total of 100 by the age of ten. There are at least 100 viruses that cause the common cold, and it would take more years than any of us get to establish immunity to each one.

Because the common cold is usually caused by a virus, no amount of antibiotics will have any effect on curing this annoying condition. I believe that antibiotics can only make matters worse. But no matter, physicians continue to prescribe certain antibiotics for relief from a cold, even though they know all too well that they won't do any good. According to the National Ambulatory Medical Care Survey (NAMCS), 110 million prescriptions for antibiotics were issued in 1992. And it has been estimated that anywhere from 18 to 60 percent of patients with colds leave their physicians offices with a prescription for an antibiotic.

So, if your child has a cold, don't rush off to the pediatrician and demand an antibiotic. If your child is offered one, ask the doctor if it is really necessary: Does he/she think your child has a bacterial infection that requires antibiotics? Or is it a viral infection that won't respond to any antibiotics? It's important to be an educated consumer, especially in the case of healthcare.

earaches

I believe that there are other medical conditions for which antibiotics are prescribed too freely. One such instance is with otitis media, without an effusion, better known as an earache. It is now clear that many cases of otitis are caused by a virus, something that is not treatable with an antibiotic. The fact is, in the absence of a painful, bulging eardrum, a child's otitis may not warrant antibiotics. And yet that is often just what physicians do prescribe.

In an interesting study published in May 1987 in *Clinical Pediatrics,* several researchers reported an association between the frequency of otitis media in early childhood and later hyperactivity. These researchers found that 69 percent of children medicated for hyperactivity had a history of more than ten ear infections, whereas only 20 percent of nonhyperactive children had that many ear infections.

This is a very significant finding, but unfortunately there have not been many follow-up investigations. Could this be because these children received too many antibiotics? The association appears significant, but there would have to be further investigations to discover the true etiology.

treatments for the common cold

There are many ways to treat winter and summer colds without using medications at all. The first thing I recommend is vitamin C (and remember, vitamin C comes in a powder form, so it is suitable for even the youngest of children). You should start with 250 milligrams every two hours until your child gets diarrhea. Once that occurs, you know you've gone too far. The next day, reduce the dosage by 500 milligrams. The next thing to do is to add garlic, 400 milligrams per day; quercetin, 240 milligrams per day; and echinacea, with or without goldenseal, one to three capsules (with the lesser amount being for the smaller child), every three hours until the symptoms start to go away. Other nutritional supplements I couldn't be without during cold and flu season are citrus bioflavonoids such as rutin and elderberry. We shouldn't forget zinc, beta-carotene, selenium, magnesium, and folic acid. I have found these to be particularly safe, with almost no overdose potential, and well tolerated in the pediatric population; I use these quite frequently and liberally with my patients.

Other common complaints that can be treated with the same regime of nutritional supplements are a sore throat and earaches. Sore throats may be the first sign of a cold, or they may be the harbinger of a more serious disease, such as strep throat. Strep throat must be treated with antibiotics because, if left untreated, it may cause serious long-lasting complications to your child's heart. Don't leave things to chance. Have your child seen by your local pediatrician. If your child's doctor says it's not strep throat, then you may be able to try some of the nutritional supplements I've outlined, and you'll be amazed at how well they usually work.

Common Cold, Flu, Earache, and Sore Throat, in Short

❖ Phase 1 diet for overweight kids

❖ Phase 2 diet if your child is not overweight

❖ Nutritional supplements as described above, including vitamin C, echinacea, zinc gluconate, citrus bioflavonoids, vitamin A, garlic, selenium, elderberry, and folic acid

sinusitis

Sinusitis is often associated with the common cold. It is something I see frequently in my adult patients, but it is becoming increasingly common in my younger patients, as well.

Sinusitis is an inflammation of the lining of the sinuses, which are the air pockets in the bones around the nose. This can be caused by the common cold, allergies, infections, cigarette smoke, or dust, among other things. This inflammation can lead to congestion and pressure in the nasal passages.

There is acute sinusitis and chronic sinusitis. Most of our children will be suffering from a chronic condition, one that is caused by irritants that are in your child's everyday environment. This is a very difficult condition to treat and even more difficult to eradicate completely. If there is a true infection present, acute sinusitis, usually typified by severe pain and dark green or yellow drainage from the nose, is a condition that is best treated by antibiotics. And remember, whenever your child takes antibiotics, he or she should also take probiotics!

In the conventional medical world, chronic sinusitis is a problem that it is often treated with repeated courses of antibiotics. Suffice it to say, this is not what I would consider the correct treatment for chronic sinusitis. In fact, in my clinical experience, it only makes the condition worse. The reason is the same as with any other condition where there is an excess of antibiotics used without good cause. This overuse of antibiotics will likely cause an overgrowth of candida. Symptoms of a yeast infection can be the same as that of chronic sinusitis. Therefore, trying to cure chronic sinusitis with more antibiotics is similar to a dog chasing its own tail.

The best treatment for chronic sinusitis is simply eliminating the source of the irritant to the sinus cavities. Easier said than done, however. To control sinusitis, you must control the triggers for the sinus irritation. You can do this by controlling the symptoms of colds and by avoiding the allergens that may trigger sinusitis in your child. For any child suffering from this condition, I would recommend a yeast-free, Phase 1 or Phase 2 diet, depending on their weight, and antiyeast supplements as previously described. Also, I would recommend flushing the sinuses with warm salt water. This is available in most pharmacies, or you can make this at home: add one-half teaspoon of salt to one cup of warm water, and stir until the salt is dissolved. Draw the saltwater solution into a dropper, place the tip about one-quarter inch into one nostril while holding the other nostril closed, and then squirt the solution and breathe through the one nostril. This can be repeated for the other nostril. Inhaling steam can also work. The child should drink plenty of fluids, as the fluid intake will help loosen the mucous so it can drain from the sinus linings.

Acute Sinusitis Treatment in Short

❖ Antibiotics

❖ Probiotics

Chronic Sinusitis Treatment in Short

❖ Phase 1 diet (yeast-free), if your child is overweight

❖ Phase 2 diet (yeast-free), if your child is not overweight

❖ Nutritional supplements as described previously

❖ Warm nasal spray or drops

Attention Deficit Disorder and Attention Deficit Hyperactivity Disorder

E VAN WAS EIGHT YEARS OLD WHEN HIS PARENTS WERE GIVEN A DIAGNOSIS of attention deficit hyperactivity disorder (ADHD) for him by his pediatrician. His parents were devastated. Evan was a child who was constantly being asked to leave the classroom because he could not control himself. He would blurt out answers, talk to the other children when his teacher was talking, and cause an overall disruption in the classroom.

Evan's parents were given a prescription for Ritalin and told that he should remain on this indefinitely. Almost as upset with that prospect as they were with the diagnosis, they believed there had to be another answer.

In Evan's case, they were right. After conducting a thorough medical history and physical examination, I ordered a cytotoxic food sensitivity test, a candida antibody test, and a glucose tolerance test along with the other routine blood tests. The results showed that Evan's blood reacted to several food products, such as corn, wheat, rye, and oats. He did not react to the candida antibody tests. The remainder of his chemistries and hematology tests were all normal.

However, his glucose tolerance test was abnormal. Evan had a severe case of hypoglycemia. In the third hour of the test (you'll recall it's a multihour test), Evan's blood sugar dropped to 38. The normal low number for the third hour is 65 to 70.

Armed with these results, I was able to outline a program for Evan. I should mention that Evan was not overweight, so I started him on Phase 2 of the Next Generation Diet in order to first correct his blood sugar imbalance. I eliminated the foods to which he had a sensitivity, and I started him on a nutritional supplementation program specifically designed for him.

In the course of the next several months, after we began the diet and nutritional supplementation program, Evan's ability to concentrate and focus improved dramatically, to the point where he was allowed to remain in the classroom the entire day. This was quite an accomplishment for a child who was being asked to leave the classroom on an almost daily basis. But perhaps even more importantly, Evan never needed to use the Ritalin that was prescribed.

attention deficit hyperactivity disorder

Attention deficit hyperactivity disorder (ADHD) or attention deficit disorder (ADD) are common neurologically based behavioral disorders affecting up to 10 percent of all school-age children. Although these two conditions are somewhat different, I use the terms interchangeably. A child with ADHD has an attention deficit or distractibility, coupled with hyperactivity or the inability to sit still, focus, or concentrate. A child who only manifests the attention deficit without the hyperactivity is given the diagnosis of ADD. ADD is the term with which most people are familiar and that is the term I will use throughout this book.

ADD is much more common in males than females in a 3:1 or a 6:1 ratio depending on the criteria used for diagnosis. The main characteristics of this disease are age-inappropriate levels of inattention, (the rule of thumb for this is whether the child can sit still as long as other children of the same age), hyperactivity, and impulsivity that manifests itself prior to the age of seven. One of the reasons so much attention is focused on this recently is because it has been found that many children with ADD turn into adults with an increased risk for mental disorders, irresponsible and impulsive lifestyles, and sociopathic behaviors.

In the decade prior to 1981, there was a 248 percent increase in the prescription of stimulant medications. Ritalin is only one of the drugs prescribed for this condition. Pemoline and dextroamphetamine are also commonly used. These drugs are prescribed because studies have shown that they result in positive effects in the child's reading and math scores, information processing, and learning ability. What the mainstream press has failed to publicize is that these benefits occur to children who have not been diagnosed with ADD but have still been given the stimulant drugs.

ritalin

Methylphenidate hydrochloride, tradename Ritalin as it is most commonly known, is the drug of choice for the treatment of ADD and is now one of the most prescribed drugs in this country. Ritalin is an amphetamine and is something I would not want my child to be taking unless it were the only solution to his problem, which I don't believe it is. Nevertheless, it is given to 10 percent of all North American boys ages six to fourteen. The International Narcotics Control Board reports ten times as much usage in the U.S. as in the rest of the world. Could American children be that much more hyperactive than the rest of the world? Are American parents simply looking for excuses for the poor behavior of their children? Or are American school teachers looking for a quick fix for the disruptions in their classrooms? I don't know if any of these are true, or even partially true. However, there must be a reason for this large discrepancy in drug usage.

The use of Ritalin is increasing at an alarming rate. Since 1980, the use of this drug has increased 125 percent in six-to-nine-year-olds and 250 percent in teenagers and adults. There are some schools in this country where one-third of all the children line up at lunchtime to take their medication. This is preposterous to me, and we need to look for other, more logical alternatives.

Ritalin, an amphetamine, is not without side effects, both physical and otherwise. The three biggest are restlessness and irritability; anorexia (meaning your child will lose his appetite possibly leading to growth disturbances); and insomnia. (Because it is an amphetamine, many children are unable to sleep when they take this medication, and this in itself may lead to learning disabilities.)

As if the physical side effects weren't enough, there are the social side effects of which the parents of many of my young patients are not even aware. If your child has ever been on Ritalin past the age of twelve, he or she will never be allowed to join the armed forces. Also, there is no way of telling how the insurance companies are going to handle this situation. ADD is a psychiatric diagnosis, carrying all of the negative connotations of one. It is entirely possible your child would be denied health insurance if they ever carried that diagnosis. No one in the medical community tells you these scenarios while they're writing out the prescription; but they should. These are very serious life complications that may arise with the simple writing of a prescription.

school ties

I can't blame the medical profession entirely for the crisis situation surrounding the increase in diagnosis of ADD. This blame has to be shared with the school system. The reason I say this is because of the typical scenario that ensues when a child is excessively disruptive in the classroom. Invariably, a teacher will write a note to the school health professional asking that the child be evaluated for ADD. The school counselor or nurse will then sit with the child for a session or two and all too often come to the decision that the child most likely has ADD. A note will then be written to the child's doctor asking that the child be evaluated for ADD. The physician, although well meaning, will generally see this note and assume that the child has ADD, without either performing or sending the child out for any psychiatric tests. The harried physician usually does this because he or she doesn't have the time to truly evaluate a child for this disorder or thinks that if the school, who sees the child a lot more often, believes the child has ADD, then it must be true. Your child is then saddled with a psychiatric diagnosis for the rest of his or her life.

There is a financial incentive for a school to have children diagnosed with ADD. For example, in New York State, the average school will receive about $8,000 in aid per year per pupil. For every child diagnosed with ADD, the amount of state aid increases to about $22,000 per student per year, a fairly sizable increase. This extra money is set aside for the hiring of school counselors and for providing extra attention for these children.

There are some schools throughout the country that have far superior ways of doing things than I've just outlined, but those schools are few and far between. So, think twice before accepting this diagnosis for your child.

is ADD a new phenomenon?

American children and young adults in the 1950s were rarely troubled by ADD. However, beginning in the late 1960s, and especially in the last decade, this diagnosis has increased tremendously, enough so that it rated a 1996 cover of *Newsweek*.

There may, in fact, be a plausible explanation as to why these disorders are being increasingly diagnosed in our children. Because of the increased awareness of this problem, many believe that it is just a matter of it coming to the attention of health officials more often. This may be part of the seeming rise in the number of young patients so diagnosed, but it simply can't account for the large overall increase seen in this disorder.

It is important not to accept a diagnosis of ADD for your child without many psychological evaluations. There are good diagnostic tools to help the clinician be sure of the recommendation, but unfortunately none of them is definitive and they are open to varying degrees of interpretation. Keep in mind that there may be other diagnoses that may account for your child's problem behavior; or there may be no diagnosis at all. For instance, it is quite ordinary to see variants in the behavior of children. Some problem behaviors can be annoying to you as an adult but still lie within the normal range for a child. Also, some poor behaviors can be the result of poor parenting or other social variables. There can even be other psychiatric conditions that are separate from ADD, such as conduct disorder or oppositional defiant disorder.

I don't mean to confuse you, but it's important that you understand that there are many factors that should and must go into the decision of labeling your child with ADD.

my child has the diagnosis— so what's a parent to do?

As a parent, the best thing you can do is to consider all treatment options before placing your child on an amphetamine such as Ritalin and make sure your child gets a proper diagnosis. The diagnosis is critical, and this is something that should take about a year to accomplish before a decision is made. There are many psychometric tests and standardized behavioral checklists that may aid in the diagnosis, but remember that nothing is definitive.

Your child needs to be evaluated by several different health professionals and interviewed with all the different caretakers present, together and then separately. We all know how differently children can behave around different authority figures.

If I suspect a child of having ADD or if a child comes to me with a diagnosis that has been properly obtained, I look at several factors that conventional medicine often overlooks, namely, the relationship among diet, the environment, and the diagnosis. I make it a point to take a detailed environmental history and to look for anything unusual and potentially toxic. This would include the type of water the child may be drinking or the amount of foods that are eaten from cans, for example. This is because an increased amount of lead has been shown to be associated with hyperactivity, and increased lead levels may be associated with contaminated drinking water or, less common these days, with eating the remnants of lead paints.

Once I've eliminated any environmental problems—and this includes food sensitivities—I recommend the Phase 1 diet for any child that needs to lose weight and the Phase 2 diet for any child who is not overweight. I also recommend that the parent feed the child foods that are as preservative-free as possible.

Ben F. Feingold, M.D., has written on the subject of diet and how it affects learning disabilities and hyperactivity. Dr. Feingold recommends a diet that contains no salicylates (aspirin, aspirin-like substances, or the natural sources of salicylates, which include tomatoes, cucumbers, apples, apricots, cherries, grapes and raisins, grape drinks, wine, nectarines, oranges, peaches, plums, prunes, and almonds) and no artificial colors or artificial flavors. If nothing else is working, I feel this is worth a try, as it is certainly far better to try this than to put your child on amphetamines.

Interestingly, in a study published in *The American Journal of Clinical Nutrition*, it was reported that there was a correlation between low omega-3 fatty acid blood levels and behaviorial problems in young boys. In a follow-up study published in *Physiology and Behavior*, the researchers more extensively observed the original group of 100 boys aged six to twelve. They found that the study participants who exhibited low levels of omega-3 fatty acids reported more physical symptoms, such as dry skin and hair, and excessive thirst. They also ranked higher in behavioral tests that gauged anxiety, hyperactivity, and impulsivity—all elements of ADD. Their parents also reported that the children in this group experienced more frequent and excessive temper tantrums, as well as problems getting to sleep and waking in the morning. For this reason, I always recommend these oils for all my patients with ADD.

Other nutritional supplements I use with my patients on a case-by-case basis include:

- ❖ St. John's wort—This is believed to work by inhibiting the re-uptake of serotonin, similar to the way an antidepressant like Prozac works. ADD may be caused by a chemical imbalance in the brain, and this may correct that imbalance.

- ❖ Phosphatidyl sereine—This is another brain neurotransmitter that may correct the neurochemical imbalance in a child's brain with ADD.

- ❖ Inositol—This may work as a mild sedative to calm the child, making him or her less likely to be inattentive or impulsive.

- ❖ GABA—This is another brain neurotransmitter that has been postulated to work in ways similar to the ones described above.

- ❖ Acetyl-l-tyrosine—This is a precursor to serotonin and has been postulated to work in similar ways to those previously described.

- ❖ Kava-kava—This is a Polynesian herb that is believed to have a calming effect and may work on some of the symptoms of ADD, similar to inositol.

other treatments for ADD

In my practice I use many different types of alternative treatments and consult with many different practitioners when I am treating a child with ADD. There are other alternatives that I would like to mention but will not be explaining in detail. These include eidetic imagery, crawling exercises, and, my personal favorite, listening to the music of Mozart. This is my favorite because the effects are almost immediate. Your child should listen to this music through headphones while he or she is doing their homework. I have found it helps the child to focus and may help to improve test scores. Another simple thing to do is to touch your child on the shoulder or hand or somewhere on the upper body while speaking to them. Again, the focus becomes much clearer, and therefore, concentration improves. There are many other simple techniques such as these that can improve your child's ADD without the harmful use of medication. I urge you to try some of these before resorting to medication.

ADD Treatment in Short

- ❖ Phase 1 or Phase 2 diet, as appropriate
- ❖ Elimination of any food sensitivities
- ❖ Nutritional supplementation, such as DMAE (di-methyl amino ethanol) in a dose of 100 to 500 milligrams per day in divided doses
- ❖ Zinc in a dose of 10 to 200 milligrams per day in divided doses
- ❖ Vitamin B complex, one to three tablets per day, in divided doses
- ❖ The oils, omega-3 in the form of borage oil and fish oils, in a dose range of 250 to 1,000 milligrams per day in divided doses; and omega-6 fatty acids in the form of GLA and flaxseed oils, in the same dosage ranges
- ❖ Behavioral techniques as described above

I have had a great deal of success with this method treating kids for ADD. It is something I discuss on the radio and lecture about quite frequently. I have found the program mentioned above quite useful, and if you're interested in some of these substances, please consult a physician in your local area knowledgeable in prescribing them.

26

Nutrients and Supplements

I'D LIKE TO SHARE A BRIEF STORY OF WHAT HAPPENED TO ME THE DAY I was writing this chapter. I received a phone call from the mother of one of my star patients, Josh. She called to tell me that Josh had experienced his first earache in one and a half years, and he was beginning to wheeze for the first time since he'd started visiting me. I suspected that Josh had been lax with both his diet and his supplement regimen for at least two weeks. My suspicions were confirmed when his mother proceeded to tell me that Josh had been feeling so well that he got lazy—a common occurrence, after feeling well for so long. They had gone on vacation, and Josh had forgotten to pack his nutritional supplements.

After feeling the effects of not having his supplements and learning how rotten it felt to be sick again, he promised never to stop taking his nutrients or to go off his diet again. By the time his mother had called,

Josh had already restarted his nutrient regimen and was beginning to feel better.

Many of my patients, after feeling better for an extended period of time, will become lax with their program. It is a very human quality, and we all do it to some extent in our lives. The program I devise for my patients is a total program. It includes diet and nutritional supplementation, and one goes hand in hand with the other. I have found they work synergistically: that is, they work even more effectively when done simultaneously.

the food chain

No matter how well you or your child might be eating, it is virtually impossible to obtain all the necessary nutrients from our food supply, simply for the reason that everything we eat has been, at one time or another, manipulated by human hands. Almost nothing we eat is in its original, unaltered state.

What I mean by this is that everything we feed the animals we eat, everything that is polluted into our atmosphere, and everything that goes into the soils where our food is grown become part of the food chain and have a profound effect on our health.

Even if we assume that the food that makes it to our kitchens is perfectly safe and nutritious because, for example, you only serve your family organic foods, then certainly it loses its value in the way we have come to prepare our foods. Most foods are either boiled too long, drawing out and eliminating any of the nutrients in the vegetable; fried in an oil that has turned rancid or has the wrong combination of essential fatty acids (this will almost always be true if you are dining out or eating any preprepared foods), overcooked; or, worse, burned, leading to an increase in free radical formation.

When meats become charred or burned, it leads to a release of methionine, which has been postulated to lead to an increased risk of heart disease by raising homocysteine levels. Interestingly enough, a nutritional supplement, folic acid, can safely and effectively bring down this homocysteine level, thus reducing your child's risk of heart disease in later life.

I believe there should be a more nutritious way of providing abundance, one that allows it to be healthy. Consumers need to demand this and then expect it to be the rule. We've become too complacent and have been led to believe that our best interests and our health have been kept in mind.

I don't believe this to be the case, and therefore we must take nutritional supplements in order to ensure our good health and especially the health of our children. There is no way children (or adults, for that matter) can possibly consume all the nutrients they need without supplementing their diet. This is especially true of the unfortunate children who are placed on a low-fat diet by their well-intentioned parents, wherein several micronutrients (vitamins and minerals) are missing. And by supplementation I mean not only vitamins, but sometimes minerals and herbals.

when is the best time to start?

Our habits are formed early, and if we can get our children to take vitamins every day, then I feel we have done a good job as parents.

Because not all of my readers can be my patients, I would like to offer some general advice that will work for nearly everyone. Nutritional supplementation may aid in treating many common disorders. As previously mentioned, I feel these nutritional supplements are generally safer and may be able to work in place of conventional medications at times, especially for the health problems I've been talking about. In this chapter, I will concentrate on the nutrients that I feel are essential to any child who either needs to lose weight or wants to stay healthy for a lifetime.

The weight-loss group of children require one list of nutrients, while the children who follow this diet simply for general health reasons have a smaller yet equally important group of nutrients. I should point out that it is completely possible to be on my diet without the use of nutritional supplements; yet, as in Josh's case, the two together can bring on a very desirable effect—better health than either one alone.

Every one of the children who come to my office is placed on a nutrient protocol best suited for him or her. Each patient is an individual and must be treated as such. On my weekly radio broadcast, listeners will call in and want to know which vitamin they should take. I will suggest the nutrient I would use in their situation, but I always caution them that they should seek the advice of a competent physician who can answer their question after making him- or herself fully familiar with their medical history.

Nutritional supplements should only be taken on the advice of a physician, not because you heard it was doing something for someone you know. The advice I offer you in this book represents the bare basics of the supplement program I would put a patient on if they were to come to my office.

The supplements I'll mention are essentially harmless to almost anyone, so I feel comfortable enough to share some of the dosages and strengths with readers that I will never meet personally. In this chapter, I will be recommending dosages of nutrients that often exceed the recommended daily allowances (RDA) determined by our government. In my experience, I have found the RDAs are often too low a dose to be effective.

calcium

The first nutrient I should mention is calcium. Because milk is restricted on this diet, many of you are probably wondering how your child's bones will grow. Let me begin by saying that I believe cow's milk is overrated as an efficient source of calcium.

Milk contains a large amount of phosphorous. This phosphorous interferes with the absorption of calcium. The average diet of most children is already too high in phosphorous because of the amount of carbonated beverages the child consumes, and this can cause a mineral imbalance and a calcium deficiency. The amount of phosphorous differs from soft drink brand to soft drink brand, and because the phosphorous content is not required on the nutrition label, it is hard to know as a consumer which one is better than the other. Suffice it to say, soft drinks are unhealthy for children.

My diet does not eliminate all dietary sources of calcium, because cheeses are still allowed. Following is a table of some common cheeses and their calcium counts.

❖ Calcium in Common Cheeses ❖

Cheese	Amount	Calcium Content (milligrams)
cottage	½ cup	140
camembert	1 ounce	150
bleu	1 ounce	150
mozzarella	1 ounce	160
cheddar	1 ounce	200
provolone	1 ounce	210
ricotta (whole milk)	½ cup	216
swiss	1 ounce	270

By comparison, an 8-ounce serving of whole milk has 290 milligrams of calcium, and 8 ounces of plain yogurt contains 400 milligrams of calcium.

Cheese is allowed on the Next Generation Diet because it does not contain sugar. During the manufacture of cheese and its fermentation process, the sugar is eliminated. Therefore, it is permissible on all phases of the diet, unless your child is on the yeast-free version.

Dark leafy vegetables, such as kale, collard greens, bok choy, and turnip greens, are excellent sources of calcium. Other foods that are great sources of calcium are sardines, mackerel, crab meat, and broccoli. If you can't get your child to eat these items, please refer to the following chart that lists the calcium contents of some common foods.

❖ Calcium Content of Common Foods ❖

Food	Amount	Calcium Content (milligrams)
VEGETABLES		
bok choy	1 cup (cooked)	250
broccoli	1 cup	190
collard greens	1 cup (cooked)	289
kale	1 cup	210
mustard greens	1 cup (cooked)	193
spinach	1 cup	200
sweet potatoes	1 medium	52
turnip greens	1 cup (cooked)	252
FISH		
bluefish	4 ounces	325
crab meat	1 cup	246
haddock	4 ounces	280
mackerel	4 ounces	300
salmon, red	4 ounces	290
sardines	4 ounces	500
scallops	4 ounces	130
shrimp	4 ounces	130
tuna	3 ounces	199
BEANS		
soybeans	1 cup (cooked)	138
tofu	¼ ounce	145
lima	1 cup	63
NUTS		
almonds	½ cup	160
pecans	½ cup	42
peanuts	½ cup	107

Because many people mistakenly believe that milk is the only dietary source of calcium, I always have my patients take a calcium supplement. I recommend calcium citrate, calcium hydroxyapatite, or calcium aspartate. I recommend a dosage of 800 to 1,500 milligrams per day in divided doses, one pill with each meal. You don't want your child to take too much calcium, otherwise you run the risk of upsetting the body's own mineral balance system. For example, if your child exceeded this recommended dosage, there may be a problem with the absorption of zinc, and your child would become deficient in that nutrient. To help the calcium get absorbed into your child's body, he or she should also be taking 250 milligrams of magnesium with each calcium tablet, and depending on the time of year and where you live, I also advise 400 IU of vitamin D_3. The vitamin D_3 should be taken by everyone who takes calcium supplements. However, it is especially important for children who live in the northeast, mid-Atlantic, Midwest, or mountain states in the months of October to April. This is the time of year when there is not enough sunlight to convert vitamin D to its active form in the body. Because calcium relies on vitamin D_3 for its uptake by the body, calcium absorption is at its lowest this time of the year. These three supplements work in tandem to help calcium get absorbed by the body.

Female adolescents especially require at least 1,200 milligrams of calcium per day (adolescent girls may also need additional iron, depending on their menstrual cycle and whether there are any menstrual-cycle irregularities; they will also require approximately 0.8 milligrams—800 micrograms—of folic acid per day).

antioxidants

Antioxidants are a necessary part of anyone's nutrient protocol. Our bodies are constantly being bombarded with free radicals that have been formed either in the foods we're eating or in something we've been exposed to environmentally. These free radicals cause cellular damage in a process known as oxidation. Antioxidants help to control some of this damage. There is much research being done now on different types of antioxidants. There are vitamin, mineral, phytochemical, and herbal antioxidants. For children, who by the very nature of their age have had less free radical exposure than adults, I recommend a small list of antioxidants that includes vitamin C, in a dose of 500 to 1,000 milligrams per day; vitamin E, in a dose of 400 IU per day; selenium, in a dose of 50 IU per day; and beta-carotene in a dose of 10,000 IU per day. These dosages can usually be obtained by taking one or two pills per day of a multiple antioxidant vitamin.

Note: At first glance, my diet might seem to be low in phytochemicals, the nutrients found in the skin and coloring of fruits and vegetables. In fact, although fruit is not a major component of this diet, the Next Generation Diet will probably have your child eating more vegetables than he or she ever has in the past.

multivitamins

Other vitamins that I feel are essential for all my patients are contained in a good multivitamin with minerals, which should contain roughly thirty or so different vitamins and minerals, including the B vitamins, zinc, manganese, and magnesium, among others. I usually recommend one or two of these tablets per day, depending upon the particular brand of vitamin supplement and what it may contain. Because the age range of children who can benefit from this book is vast, it's hard to recommend so many different doses for so many different vitamins and minerals.

weight-buster supplements

In my experience, there are at least two nutritional supplements essential for losing weight. The first is chromium, which is thought to help regulate the secretion of insulin and hence the metabolism of sugar. Chromium is a key nutrient in any dieter's program, adults or children. It can be taken in the picolinate or polynicotinate variety. The only difference between the two is a slight change in the molecule that makes one more absorbable for some patients than others.

There was some controversy surrounding chromium. In doses that exceed what humans ingest by 6,000 percent, some laboratory rats got cancer. However, there is no other source of chromium in the American diet other than by nutritional supplementation. It is not found in our soil, where we get so many of our other nutrients. Therefore, if you want it in your child's diet, it must be taken in the form of a pill.

If you are providing your child with supplements solely on the advice of this book, then I would recommend whichever one is available at your local health food store. The dose should be 50 to 200 micrograms three times per day.*

The other vitamin supplement I recommend for my dieters is an amino acid known as L-glutamine. It is not an essential vitamin because I find most of my weight-loss patients can get along without it, but it is especially effective for my patients who are having sugar cravings. Your child can take this at a dose of 250 milligrams to 500 milligrams, as needed, up to six to eight times per day.

I don't generally like to give children pills as an answer to a sugar craving because of the psychological implications of taking a pill to handle a problem. It would be best if your child could learn to deal with the sugar craving in a more constructive way. One thing I have found that works really well when a craving hits, before acting on impulse, is to sit back and take deep breaths for five minutes. An adult or older child can use this time to analyze the situation that created the food craving. Was it stress? Sadness? Joy? This can help your child to understand why he or she is having food cravings. Is it because they are hungry, or is it something else? If it's something else, this is just the kind of the behavior we are trying to change.

A younger child can just take a "time out." The sugar craving will most likely pass after the five minutes are over. If it doesn't, then your child will be able to get a snack that is permitted on the diet, and the impulsiveness of the behavior is diminished. Eating should never be done impulsively, and this is the lesson your child needs to learn. However, in the toughest cases, I have found L-glutamine to be a very helpful addition to a daily vitamin regimen.

There are many other nutritional supplements I recommend to my patients on a daily basis. The ones I've outlined here are the bare essentials most children should be taking.

---

* In this book, I have provided dosage ranges. Remember, every child is an individual and their nutrient regimen would have to be planned accordingly. The guideline I use is usually weight, not age. I have known some ten-year-olds who weigh as much as I do. So, if your child is lower on the scale, then use the lower doses that I recommend, If they weigh more, then the higher doses would most likely fit your child's needs. This is not an exact science, and so I often have to adjust my patient's nutrients at each visit, depending upon the particular need at the time.

27

Shaping the Future

HOLIDAYS WERE AN AMAZING FOOD EXPERIENCE IN MY HOUSEHOLD when I was growing up. A typical holiday meal would consist of a cold antipasto, a warm antipasto, the pasta course and then a meat course with vegetables and other starches, followed two or more hours later (we needed room to digest all this food) by several dessert choices. To this day, I cannot cook a meal for exactly the number of people coming to dinner. It always looks as if five times the number is joining me.

Allow your child to make his or her own food choices, but from what you have to offer. Don't force them or expect them to eat everything you've made. This is every bit as important as any other value you instill in your child. As a parent, *you* are the role model. You can't simply abdicate your responsibility by adhering to the philosophy of "do as I say, not as I do." Success in this weight loss/healthy nutritional lifestyle endeavor will increase if all family members change the way they eat and increase their exercise.

One excellent way to approach this problem before it's too late is to assess your child's weight before puberty. If he or she is overweight, do something about it immediately. Weight is not a problem that will go away of its own accord. Besides, younger children are far more apt to be receptive to taking advice. It is be a good idea to at least offer them the kind of advice they need to lose weight in a healthy fashion, rather than having them learn it on the street or, even worse, from television or to make it up themselves, as I did when I was young. There are, to my mind, far too many horrible images gleaned from television to allow it to be the source of nutrition education. Instead, let's teach them the right way to eat.

who should be part of this diet?

Other members of the family who need to be involved in the Next Generation Diet are the ones doing the grocery shopping and the meal preparation. This can include older siblings, grandparents, or household help. Have them read the book, too.

how to keep all ages on the diet

Six-to-Eight-year-olds

Six-to-eight-year-olds may have problems in social situations, but their problems will generally have to be handled by you. You must identify all the potential hardships and talk to your children about the situation, not as a problem but in a matter-of-fact way. They will think there is nothing unusual about the circumstances unless you give them an impression that there is. For example, they are often unaware that bringing different foods to a party is unusual unless you make it seem that way. This age group tends to obey their parents with more regularity than the other two, so you can take advantage of this.

Nine-to-Twelve-year-olds

The nine-to-twelve-year-olds often have ideas of what they want to eat. This is healthy and not the main problem. They assert some independence, but with much less rigor than teenagers. For most of these kids, the biggest problem for them remains what to eat in social situations without feeling like an outsider. It's very important for them to have a social identity and for them not to be considered "different" or "odd" by their peers. Ask your child to identify these social situations, whether it be a cupcake party at school, or a "sleep-over" at a friend's home, and work together to form a solution. There is always a solution, and this is an important concept for your children to understand. If you feel a solution can be found for any problem, so will they.

Teenagers

Unless a teenager is involved in all aspects of the diet, I can almost guarantee that it will not succeed. I'm not saying that they have to like what they're going to be doing, but they should feel that they are a part of it and that it's not being forced on them from on high. As a rule, teenagers hate being told what to do. They have to want to do this for themselves. I lost weight as a teenager only because I wanted to, not because I was forced to.

Once you've completed their food diary, it's important to let them see what's wrong with their diet. I often recommend allowing the teen to do the circling of the food that they might suspect is not part of this new nutritional plan on their own, and then you can review it with them later.

Set reasonable goals. Encourage and emphasize the notion that all humans do not and should not look alike; that there are often genetic differences that will prevent your daughter from ever looking like the waiflike models posing in the fashion magazines; and that your son may never be able to resemble some of his favorite sports or film heroes because of genetics. But this is not a tragedy. Emphasize that it is variety and differences that enable the world to be a more interesting place in which to live.

Don't be afraid to ask your teenager what he or she had to eat that day. However, don't make a big issue over some small indiscretion because you don't want to turn them off the idea of dieting. Instead of asking a general question such as, "What did you have to eat today?" ask, "What vegetables did you have to eat today?" or "How was that chicken salad I made for you?" This way, you will get the information you want while avoiding the potential for confrontation.

Stock your shelves at home only with foods permitted on the diet. Most children eat at least two meals at home, and teenagers especially do a lot of snacking. If you only have the foods he or she can eat, then two-thirds of the battle is won. Even if you aren't there all the time to personally prepare the food, if you know what food is in the house, you'll know that your child will be eating right.

picky eaters

It's not unusual for a child to complain about the food you serve and then refuse to eat it. Twelve-year-old girls are notorious for trying to exert their independence from their parents by using food as a weapon. This is a common age for eating disorders such as anorexia or bulimia to manifest themselves. At this age, girls will often eat in a way that is the exact opposite of how they've always eaten. They are looking for some-thing to call their own.

If your children will not eat what you've offered and if they cannot behave properly at the dinner table, my advice is to just ask them to leave the room and to sit quietly until they are prepared to eat what you've served. Don't get angry, and don't make a fuss. This is a lot eas-ier to say than actually do, but it is your most effective weapon against this kind of behavior. Do not allow them back to the dinner table for dessert, and *don't* let them eat anything until the next mealtime. This is the way my parents handled me, and, nutritionally speaking, it was probably one of the best things they ever did for me. I'm not saying you should be extremely rigid in what you serve. Quite the contrary. Try to serve something your child would like to eat, but don't turn your-self into a short-order cook. If your child doesn't like what's served, then the kitchen is closed. And don't be afraid to stand your ground. Believe me, your child won't starve. Plenty of times I walked away from the table without eating anything, and it certainly didn't adversely affect my health in any way. What it did do was to teach me respect for my parents and their wishes.

If you are prepared to be a short-order cook, then cook only what is on their diet. Make sure the right foods are always available.

I know it may seem harsh, but children will test you with bad behavior. If you give in to them once, it is impossible to reverse the momentum. Any child psychologist will tell you that children are trying to expand their universe at all times, and as unpleasant as this may be to contemplate, this includes their relationship with their parents.

Some children get fixated on one particular food. If this is a problem, just make sure that you serve different types of foods at each meal. Eventually, your child will come around. If you make too much of this behavior, it will only reinforce it, and your child will continue to do this over and over. But I suggest that you try to avoid this confrontation by allowing your child this small indiscretion so long as it is not harmful—I would not want your child to eat only chocolate pudding, or french fries, for example!

Some children will eat only foods of a certain color. Don't treat this as a problem by trying to force feed foods of other colors. But do offer foods of other colors to your child. If he doesn't want them, do not acknowledge this at all. Just keep going about your normal routine without so much as a raised eyebrow. Trust me, eventually your child will move on. I have often found that if this behavior of eating only one color of food is reinforced by all the focus on it at mealtime, it will only serve to further encourage such behavior.

talking about food

I always recommend that the television be turned off at mealtimes. I find it to be a terrible distraction for younger children. Mealtimes should be quality time spent together as a family. And if the television is turned off, this will prove to your child that you take mealtimes very seriously. It will begin to make your child understand that eating is more than just sustenance.

Meals are about nutrition, and it's not a bad idea to spend time talking about this at the dinner table. I often recommend that the parents of my patients spend some time discussing what they are eating and why. However, at the same time you're trying to educate, you should also try to make it a fun experience for your child. For example, why not explain to your child why you've chosen to serve brown rice instead of mashed potatoes. Initially, at least, this will help reinforce the changes you've made in the family's eating habits. Additionally, it will serve to emphasize the importance of a healthy balanced diet.

keeping your child on the straight and narrow

Unless you're willing to hire a food detective to follow your child around all day, you must have faith that your child is going to behave in the same fashion as you would expect him or her to behave in your presence. For instance, if your child is well-mannered around you, there's a good chance he or she will display the same behavior when you're not around. If eating and nutrition is given importance in the hierarchy of what you teach your children, then this should not be a problem when you're not the one providing the meal.

We sometimes forget that table manners are only a small part of what we must teach our children concerning food and nutrition. Too often we let them get away with things we would never permit in any other part of their growth. We tolerate them eating only certain foods or watching television during mealtimes, yet we would never let them get away with allowing them to choose when they want to do their homework. Granted, homework is not the same as choosing not to eat broccoli, yet the behavioral standard should be the same. Doing your homework will be beneficial to you as an adult, and so will eating correctly. Spend time teaching good nutrition.

problem times

There are three main areas that all parents perceive as problems for dieting: parties, school days, and sleep-away or day camp. It is relatively easy to allow your child to enjoy these activities while still staying on the diet. Remember, for the child who needs to lose weight, this is not a diet that will ostracize him, and for the nonoverweight child, it is nothing more than a balanced, healthy diet. I don't want your child to feel singled out or different, and one look at the menu ideas will show you how true that is.

Parties

Let's start with parties, probably the easiest situation to deal with. Call the mother who is throwing the party and find out what the menu is going to be. If it is going to be the typical American child's birthday party, there is sure to be an assortment of sugar in all its forms: cake, candy, and ice cream. If this is the case, then explain the situation to the other parent and ask if it would be okay to send along a special party snack. I had one patient's mother send over my strawberry and cream frozen dessert and some yam chips (see the recipe section for the first of these items). These created quite a stir. Instead of feeling like an outsider as his mother had feared, her son became the hit of the party. Fortunately, she had sent over more than enough for her son, and he was able to share with his friends. The next day, my patient's mother received several phone calls asking for the recipe for the dessert and snacks she had prepared. It was the first time the parents of her son's friends had seen her son since he'd been on a diet. As it happened, they were very impressed with the weight loss he was achieving and the types of foods he was allowed to eat while maintaining this weight loss.

The hard-and-fast rule for this situation is to prepare in advance. Make a few phone calls to the person in charge of the event. It doesn't matter whether the party is in a private home, a school, or a restaurant. My advice is the same: send along something. The beauty of this diet is that the food you send will be very similar to the foods that are already there, only prepared in a more healthy fashion.

School Days

As for school lunches, I generally recommend that your children take to school the lunches you have prepared for them. This is the only way to ensure that you know what they are eating. Besides, it will almost always be something healthier and fresher than what would be on the school menu. Preparing food in a healthy way tends to be a little more costly than usual because you are often using fresher and therefore more expensive ingredients—in the long run, however, these few extra pennies a day may protect the health of your family.

As a grade schooler, I always took my lunch from home, and I always thought that the kids who ate from the school cafeteria were cooler. Your task is to make this not so with your child by making lunch from home seem natural and better tasting. Don't make it seem like an effort to make the lunch. Try and make it the night before and make it together with your child having the most input. You can do this by making a separate shopping day, or a separate part of the normal shopping trip, devoted solely to school lunches that your child can help choose. The trick is to enroll your child into this diet by making him or her think they have a lot of say into what they are eating.

If you pack the food in containers, you won't need sandwiches. Make a prepared lunch seem more exotic than a school lunch. To that end, make sure it's packed in a colorful container. For the younger kids, include funny colored napkins. Look for different vegetables to make it more exciting.

If you refer to the recipe section, you'll find some of the great desserts you can make for your child's school lunch box.

If your child insists on buying food at school, try reviewing the school menu with them. Then, together choose the healthier foods from that school lunch menu that are part of the diet. First, let them choose, and then you can correct their choices by way of suggestions. If the school does not provide a preselected menu plan for the week, then ask your child some nonthreatening questions as I previously described about what their meal was like. You can get a lot of information from these questions without seeming as if you're prying.

As far as snacks are concerned, if you have only the foods in the house that are allowed on the diet, then your child will only have good foods to choose from. If you're concerned with them buying snacks that you don't provide, try this: when you're in the supermarket or when you take the food out of the shopping bags, openly discuss with your child which foods are good and which are not so healthy. This will help reinforce the foods that are on the diet. Encourage them to read nutrition labels and to find foods that fit the parameters of their diet before you can. Make it a contest with the reward for the most innovative menu idea being something other than food, perhaps a movie, or a trip to the mall, or some outdoor activity your child likes—something that's good for them as well.

Another word of advice: try to plan out your child's day. For instance, if your child has soccer practice after school and you know that the team always stops at Johnny's house for a snack before or after practice, then you can use the same trick I use for children attending parties. If the team always stops at a certain store to buy snacks, I would suggest going to that store beforehand and looking through the inventory to see if you and your child can find any foods that are on the diet. This way, there will be no surprises, and your child can't use the excuse that they didn't know what they could get. Again, by doing this you are allowing your child to take an active role in his or her dietary choices.

The key is to be prepared. Think ahead. I always have parents visualize their child's days. This helps identify all the trouble spots. Since you are getting the diet from this book, and I will not be there to advise you, I suggest you make an activity chart, not unlike the food diary, for a week prior to starting the diet. You can then see not only what your child is eating, but where. This will help make it infinitely easier to plan out a day's menu. It's easier for many children to have things mapped out for them. The truth is, spontaneity is far more of an adult issue than an issue for your kids. Children find comfort and security in a structured environment, and that will certainly help them stay on the diet, especially in the beginning.

Nobody's perfect, and I'm not going to be with you every step of the way, nor do I know the million and one scenarios you and your kids can get involved with in the course of a day. I simply offer these tips as suggestions. They will need to be modified according to your particular lifestyle. The diet will still work even if you don't follow any of these suggestions. All I ask is that you spend just a few minutes each week thinking about the diet and planning for it in a more organized way than you might be used to. Again, this reinforces the notion that nutrition is something to be taken seriously. We need to disinvent the fast food mentality that is so pervasive today. If we don't look out for the safety and nutritional benefits of what we're eating, no one else will. It's time we took some control over our food supply. This can be accomplished if we start one household at a time.

Camp

Many of my young patients attend camp during the summer months, whether it's sleep-away or day camp. The problem will be the same: compliance.

The trick I've found to work best is to speak to the camp counselors and the cooks at the camp. Again, the key idea is planning ahead. The cooks, or at least the administration of the camp, will more than likely know what the upcoming menus will look like. See if you can get a copy of the menus, and then try to review them with your child so there will be no surprises. Discuss what he or she should and should not eat. This is an amazing opportunity for you and your child to get more involved with each other on a different level. By being involved in the decision making, your child will feel as if he or she is being treated more as an adult. Believe me, this raises compliance levels through the roof.

Perhaps the best advice I can offer concerning camps is to start the diet several weeks prior to your child going away. This suggestion isn't nearly as important for those going to day camp because you and your child will be sharing several meals a day anyway. But it is more important to get your child who is going to sleep-away camp into a routine before leaving. This way, it will be easier for your child to stay on the diet. We are looking to set up new habits and patterns, and this is so much easier if there is a few weeks' lead time to reinforce the behaviors.

Remember, we are striving for a lifetime of success, and I want you and your child to understand that this diet is forever. It's the best opportunity you will have to provide your child with the foundation necessary for a lifetime of good health.

what to do if your child is not losing weight

First, make sure your child is following the instructions of the diet. This doesn't necessarily mean your child is cheating deliberately, so you may have to conduct an investigation. Don't come out and ask your child if he or she is cheating. Instead, seek information in a nonconfrontational way. For instance, ask, "What did you have for lunch today?" or "Did you stop off anywhere on the way home from school today?"

If the answers are dietetically correct, then you'll need to start looking for hidden sugars. As I've explained earlier, sugar is in most of the food we buy today, so you'll need to go over everything your child may be eating and look for any hidden problems. Create another food diary and double-check all the ingredients. Here's an example, which doesn't necessarily pertain to children, but it will show you what I mean: most balsamic vinegar is not permitted on the diet because it contains sugar. Most other vinegars do not. Catsup is not permitted on the diet.

This may not seem like a large incursion, but some catsups may contain as much if not more sugar than a candy bar. Inspect labels carefully, and closely examine the snack foods your child is eating, which is probably where the problem lies.

The biggest problem most children will encounter on the weight loss part of this diet has to do with their metabolism. In this book, I've outlined a diet that will work most effectively in the majority of cases. Obviously, there are going to be some children who fail on this diet plan. Having seen such cases, I have found that it usually has to do with the child's metabolism rate. Because of this, some children will have to eat fewer grams of carbohydrates than what I've outlined for their age group. For example, if you have an overweight eight-year-old and you start him or her on the diet eating 60 grams of carbohydrates a day and they're not losing weight, then you need to lower the amount of carbohydrate by 10 grams per day until you find the perfect amount that will allow for weight loss.

In addition, there are several ways to enhance your child's metabolism. The first thing to try is exercise. (In Part 4, I will offer some examples of fun exercise programs for the entire family.) If your child is like the normal American child, he or she is probably spending three or four hours a day in front of the television set or a computer screen. Obviously, this doesn't leave much time for physical activity. This has to be changed. The less active your child is, the lower his or her metabolic rate, which results in a lower amount of carbohydrates he or she can consume and still lose weight on this diet.

nutritional supplements

There are other supplements that I believe have an ability to up-regulate or increase your child's metabolism. The first one I add is L-carnitine. This is an amino acid that has some ability to increase the metabolism of the body. I usually start with 250 milligrams once a day, in the morning before meals, and increase it as necessary. You should probably, depending on the weight of your child, never exceed 3,000 milligrams per day or 1,000 milligrams at each meal. This dose would only be advisable for overweight children who weigh as much as nonoverweight adults.

Another supplement I use is ginkgo biloba, an herb. I recommend a dose of 40 milligrams per day in divided doses for the six-to-eight-year-old group and increase this to as much as 80 milligrams three times per day, depending on the age and size of your child.

I have also used co-enzyme Q10 in a dose of 30 to 90 milligrams per day to help increase a child's metabolism and to encourage faster weight loss. There are many other supplements for this purpose, too.

Try one of these if your child's weight loss has slowed or come to a halt. But don't force things or expect a rapid weight loss each week of the diet. Your child's body needs to adjust to all the changes, both physically and psychologically. This diet is not a race against time, and you should not set up expectations for your child's weight loss that may be impossible to achieve or maintain. Each child's weight loss will occur at an individual pace. You can generally expect a loss of 1 to 4 pounds a week, depending on the circumstances.

There are many potential pitfalls to any diet plan. There will probably be backsliding along the way, too. The key is not to get discouraged. Your child generally takes his clues from you. You are the team leader. If you stay enthusiastic, they will, too. With this program, I am asking you and your family to make some enormous changes. It's going to take some time. Be prepared—and be patient.

the Healthy

Fitness Zone

Couch Potatoes
Start as
Little Spuds

As an overweight child, I remember despising one of the things that could have helped rescue me from that fate — exercise. Unfortunately, I did not appreciate physical exercise until much later in life, when I was an adult and already nonoverweight. I always wonder how much easier it might have been to maintain my thinner weight had exercise been a part of my life since I was a child.

To be perfectly fair, some exercise was encouraged by my parents, but it was in the form of organized sports. I hated organized sports because, as an overweight child, I was never good enough. I was always out of breath, always placed in the worst position on the team, or worse yet, not chosen at all, forced to sit on the sidelines while all the other players seemed to be having the time of their lives. In fact, the only times I was allowed on the field or the court was because there was a rule that all children on the team had to have some playing time. You can imagine how that made me feel, and what it did for my self-esteem.

It was only as an adult, when the nautilus and "belonging to the gym" craze began, that I began to appreciate and enjoy exercise. This was something I could do on my own and compete solely with myself. I could challenge myself to go faster on the treadmill, to lift a heavier weight, and no one would know about this except me. This was a liberating experience, and I came to truly love exercise. I'm not perfect, and after a long day at the office, it takes all my strength to get to the gym; but I go and have reaped the benefits.

When I am on the gym regimen I prefer, I don't have to watch my weight. My HDL cholesterol (the good cholesterol) has never been better. I never use the elevator at our nine-story office building, and time permitting, I can run five miles without being out of breath. I could not do any of these things as a teenager, yet I can do them with ease as a thirty-five-year-old. If only I had known about these things as a kid.

the importance of exercise

Although the diet I've outlined in the previous chapters will allow your child to lose weight whether or not he or she exercises, exercise is an integral part of any overall health plan.

Exercise is important for the entire family, not just your overweight child. Exercise should be ongoing and lifelong in order for its benefits to be truly realized. As with nutrition, it must be learned early and reinforced as often as possible. Even if your child is extremely productive with the time spent in front of the computer, there simply must be time for physical activity.

To prevent obesity and the poor health outcomes associated with obesity, such as heart disease and diabetes, we need to be promoting healthful behavior that involves the entire family. This will not only foster teamwork and camaraderie, but it will avoid the stigmatization and the singling out of the overweight child. Family-oriented interventions that promote an active rather than a sedentary lifestyle need to be introduced. For example, instead of having a family outing to the movies, where everyone will be sitting for several hours eating all sorts of bad foods, go bowling or play miniature golf instead.

We live in an age when most children do not romp around outside for hours on end after school as they once might have a generation ago. This is partially a safety issue; many parents would not like to see their children playing in unattended areas. But also, many parents are more active, and many more children come from two-parent (or one-parent) working households. It is often safer for the child to be inside, where they can be more easily supervised.

By preschool age, too many of our children are already addicted to television. Is this our fault or theirs? It's probably a combination of the two. Let's examine our behavior. All too often we use television or computers as an easy baby-sitter. How many parents put on a video for their children so that they will sit quietly and watch it? We're all guilty of this, at least occasionally. The child of one of my best friends is four years old, and there is an hour-long video that she can recite word for word. I don't think this is such an uncommon occurrence.

I'm not faulting parents who do this. It's often an economic necessity for both parents to be out of the house or, in the case of one-parent families, for that parent to hold down more than one job to pay all the bills. All I'm saying is that we must examine our behavior if we are going to succeed in giving our children the nutritional lifestyle plan they need to have to survive in today's world.

If you're a couch potato, chances are good your kids will be, too. Your child will not realize that your inactivity doesn't have to be the norm. In the early, formative years, children strive to be just like their parents. They need a good example. Unfortunately, they're not getting it because over 25 percent of all American adults never exercise. This must be one of the major reasons for the decline of physical education among our children.

how much exercise do our children need?

The amount of physical activity I'm talking about does not have to be overwhelming. Exercise physiologists have begun to realize that moderate physical activity that is sustainable has as many health benefits as more vigorous physical activity for short periods of time. In recent years, we have begun to move away from the vigorous, often unattainable goals of the aerobic era to something that is far more achievable for the average person.

The first ever Surgeon General's report on Physical Activity and Health released on July 11, 1996, concluded that regular, moderate, physical activity can substantially reduce the risk of developing or dying from heart disease, diabetes, colon cancer, and high blood pressure. The report defines moderate physical activity as that which uses 150 calories of energy per day, or 1,000 calories per week. Some examples of this include walking briskly for 30 minutes, swimming laps for 20 minutes, washing and waxing a car for 45 to 60 minutes, or pushing a stroller 1½ miles in 30 minutes.

For children, this standard seems ridiculously easy to reach.

❖ Kid Friendly Exercises That Expend 150 Calories ❖

Playing volleyball for 45 minutes

Playing touch football for 30 to 45 minutes

Walking on a treadmill for 1 mile in 20 minutes

Shooting baskets for 20 minutes

Bicycling 5 miles in 30 minutes or 4 miles in 15 minutes

Fast dancing for 30 minutes

Water aerobics for 30 minutes

Playing basketball or soccer for 15-20 minutes

Jumping rope for 15 minutes

Running 1½ miles in 15 minutes

Stair walking for 15 minutes

Playing baseball for 45 minutes

The report also noted that regular participation in physical activity appeared to reduce symptoms of depression and anxiety, improve mood, and enhance the ability to perform daily tasks.

If exercise is so good for you, why isn't everyone doing it? With all the television commercials and lucrative endorsement deals for many sports figures, one would think everyone was exercising. You would also think these sports heroes would make great role models, providing an inspiration and acting as a goal for your child to attain. Not only is this far from true, but the actual figures concerning those who exercise in this country will astonish you.

According to the report, among young people aged 12 to 21, almost 50 percent are not vigorously active on a regular basis. And if you think things get better as preteens become teenagers, think again. Physical activity actually declines dramatically with age during adolescence. Only 19 percent of all high school students are physically active for 20 minutes or more in physical education classes every day during the school week, and female adolescents are much less physically active than their male counterparts. Is it any wonder that our children are getting larger and larger?

The same report went on to add that high school students' enrollment in daily physical education classes dropped from 42 percent in 1991 to 25 percent in 1995. I remember hating gym class for many reasons, the biggest being how overweight I was. Yet, it was mandatory.

One of the reasons for the decline in physical education programs for our children is the lack of its importance in the lives of the adults who are making the curriculum decisions. Another reason is a lack of adequate funding. This sad state of affairs is due to the tremendous competition in the school budget by programs for money, and all too often, it is the physical education program that is the loser. This inevitably sets the child up to believe that physical education is not important and is little more than a secondary goal. If our children are taught that physical fitness is not a top priority, this unfortunate belief can be carried with them for life.

"I'm not good enough"

I loathed my physical education classes not only because I was overweight and ashamed but because I was never good enough. The standards were high and therefore attainable by only a select few of the students. Those who did attain these goals quite naturally lauded it over those of us who did not. How many of you can remember the President's Fitness Award? I can recall thinking what a failure I was because I could never even get close to the lofty goals set by this organization. But today there has been a change in the standards set by physical education teachers. They no longer rely on performance-based standards because it was found that these benchmarks ensure that all but a handful of students fail. These new standards should help prevent our children from feeling like failures. There will always be some children who are better at certain things than others. However, if a child is judged against him- or herself, we can remove one very large obstacle in the road to physical fitness.

The National Association for Sport and Physical Education recommends the establishment of a "healthy fitness zone" that many children will be able to attain. This healthy fitness zone is a range of goals that takes into account many variations, including different skill levels. It is designed so most children will fall into one of these zones and so no one is left out. Your child will be able to maintain a level of self-esteem with these zones that was not possible years ago when everyone met one standard or failed. It is important for your child to understand that it is not necessary to be an Olympic athlete to be a healthy person and enjoy the benefits of exercise.

In order to ensure that children get the most out of their physical education experience, some schools are relying on noncompetitive activities that measure heart rates, not the speed of the fastest child.

And in some schools, selection of teams is now randomly done by computer! This eliminates one of the cruelest things that can ever happen to an overweight or nonathletic child: being chosen last or not at all. I wish they had computers to do that when I was suffering all that humiliation.

who's responsible for my child getting physical activity?

Ultimately the responsibility for the health and welfare of any child belongs to the parent. Nevertheless, the school can play a tremendous role in fostering good health. Organized education has the opportunity, mechanisms, and sometimes even the personnel to deliver nutrition education and fitness activities.

However, the proper steps taken in school are not enough to promote good health. It is absolutely necessary for the home environment to accurately reflect the changes you wish to make in the lifestyle of your children. It is not enough to rely on the school.

the benefits of exercise

In a study published in the *American Journal of Clinical Nutrition*, it was shown that in obese boys, a regimented physical training program led to an appreciable augmentation in the overall energy expenditure of these children, even with a lack of change in spontaneous physical activity. This means that even though these obese children did no additional physical activity other than their prescribed regimen, the amount of calories they used in their same daily activities increased, something every dieter hopes to achieve. These boys were able to up-regulate their metabolism — in essence, speed it up. This is not the only benefit derived from exercise. Exercise has a profound effect on your child's health.

The health of our population is moving away from acute illness to chronic illness. By this I mean that medicine is now able to treat quite effectively many of the emergency-type problems that arise. However, modern medicine is having a harder time trying to treat all the chronic illnesses, such as diabetes, heart disease, and obesity, all of which are becoming increasingly prevalent in our children — and all of which are diet-related illnesses.

For these problems, exercise works very well. In my experience, it can decrease the amount of insulin a diabetic uses and can free people with high blood pressure from medication. Steven Blair of the Cooper Institute for Aerobics Research in Dallas, one of the nation's most influential exercise scientists, reports that among people with the same illness, exercisers will live the longest and have the best outcomes.

how does exercise work?

Exercise works in two ways. The first is through strength training, and the second is through aerobic fitness. In strength training, the body adds bulk to muscle cells. Larger muscles process oxygen more efficiently, so the heart does not have to pump as hard to keep them supplied with the same amount of oxygen. This is why this type of activity is encouraged for heart patients.

Secondly, aerobic activity prompts the release of certain hormones that combat disease. For example, hypertension (high blood pressure) may be exacerbated by the body releasing from the adrenal glands too much adrenaline, in response to threatening stimuli. This response causes the heart to race and brings sugar into the bloodstream as a source of quick food for the muscles. This excess adrenaline will also raise the blood pressure above normal. With aerobic activity, the muscles become more efficient at processing the sugar and the hormones, in turn causing the adrenal glands to secrete less of these hormones in what is called a negative feedback loop.

Aerobic activity can also charge up the immune system. In response to the stress of physical activity, the body releases adrenaline and cortisol. These two hormones act to release the T cells (an important immune-system component) from the bones and the spleen, where they are stored, into the bloodstream, where they help to defend the body from invaders.

Exercise plays a role in many areas of your child's development, both physically and emotionally. Devote some real attention to it when you're raising your child. If you are anything like my parents and know nothing about exercise or what can be done, the next chapter will help you to help your child benefit from the healthy effects of exercise.

Demystifying
Exercise

Let's not forget that our children's behaviors and quite often their temperament are shaped by adult attitudes. This is an extremely important point because when it comes to organized sporting activities, it is adults who are doing the organization. Anyone who has ever watched competitive sporting events among children can attest to some of the following behaviors: kids not shaking hands with the opposing team after a close game; young athletes throwing equipment when things don't go the right way; youngsters verbally abusing teammates, coaches, or referees.

This inability to control temper and emotions in the heat of a game has a lot to do with parental pressure and other adult attitudes that place the focus on winning at all costs or avoiding a loss at all costs. Allowing this and sometimes even tacitly encouraging it, we create a situation in which our children are becoming overcompetitive.

We must create more realistic expectations for ourselves and for our children. This is important because it will aid in the whole dieting process for your overweight child and in the entire healthy eating patterns you want to establish for your nonoverweight child. Goals should be set in a realistic manner. You can't expect a five-pound weight loss every week, and the set goal should not reflect this. You *can* expect a gradual but steady weight loss over time. Expecting too much would set your child up for failure and would ultimately sabotage the whole plan.

Exercise should and will raise self-esteem. When it fails to do that, we have defeated the purpose. I know that as an overweight child myself, I could certainly have used a boost in the self-esteem department. I was ridiculed by other children because of my size and my inability to perform. It would have been healthy for my psyche had I been exposed to some form of formal exercise training at the request of my parents, exercise training that didn't fall under the category of competition. The truth was, they just didn't know what to do. I certainly don't blame them for this; it is a common problem shared by many in their generation that I want the next generation to avoid.

making exercise fun

First of all, be creative. Our busy schedules and the busy schedules of our children demand this. Set aside a specific time, at first, a few minutes a day, as exercise time. I always start my most sedentary patients on no more than five minutes of activity a day. What this does is to create a pattern or a habit of exercise being a part of daily living, not unlike the ritual of brushing your teeth every morning and every evening.

I recommend involving the entire family and as many friends as possible. This can keep exercise both distracting and fun, without detracting from valued time. Not only are you doing something good for your mental and physical health, but your child (and you) gets to spend quality time with the people they enjoy being with the most.

If you believe a gym is the best answer, be inventive and try to bargain for a family discount from your local gym. I've had many patients successfully do this. If the entire family is willing to participate in an exercise program, it may be less expensive to purchase some exercise equipment for the home, rather than pay individual fees for a gym. The equipment doesn't have to cost a lot. I've had many patients find good used gym equipment at yard sales because so many people buy equipment and abandon it. There are even resale stores for used exercise equipment.

Look for ways to turn weekend activities or vacation time into exercise. This can be as simple as parking the car in the farthest spot from the entrance to the mall and walking vigorously to it. Instead of simply taking your child to a sporting event, fan their enthusiasm for the event by recreating a miniversion of it before you actually go. Or exercise can be as complex as organizing a family canoeing trip or a hike into a nearby park or forest. Vacations can be fun if you bring the exercise along.

Unfortunately, I have far too many patients tell me that they did not exercise on their vacations. Vacation doesn't mean that you take a holiday from good health. This is a bad attitude to convey to our children. Exercise must be a part of our daily lives. No matter where you are vacationing, there is no reason that some form of regimented physical activity shouldn't take place.

With children, most of us know this is almost guaranteed to happen because whether the vacation is to a beach, a city, or another locale, there is so much extra walking and sightseeing involved that you can't help but exercise more, or at least expend more energy.

I encourage you to keep a list of fun activities the whole family can enjoy and from which they can benefit. This can be fun and an interesting challenge.

You'd be amazed at all the opportunities that arise from just slightly adjusting our daily rituals. For example, a couple of years ago, I used to take a cab home from my office every day. I decided to add exercise to this simple ritual by walking home instead. Living in Manhattan, this also made for a great opportunity to see shop windows, street fairs, and so on, that I would have overlooked by getting into a cab every day. Walking home is now something I look forward to because I never know what I'm going to see along the way.

Everyday things can become fun and provide much needed exercise. For instance, a 1993 study of college-age women found that simply walking up stairs delivered the same aerobic benefits as running on a flat surface. Since reading that study, I have encouraged my patients, young and old alike, to use the stairs at their office, to go up and down the stairs in their home, and so on. This basic exercise can be done almost anywhere and anytime, including the local mall, library, train station, or home. To do this, beginners should start out by going up and down half flights of stairs. Going down gives your lungs a brief rest. Your child shouldn't go so fast as to be gasping for air. If that happens, stop all activity, count to 30, and then resume. Your child should also stand up straight and not lean over. The lean puts too much strain on the back and may lead to injuries.

setting realistic goals

Setting realistic and attainable goals is an essential component of any diet-and-exercise plan. I am more apt to encourage the setting of exercise goals than in setting weight goals. In this way, more emphasis is placed on a positive achievement rather than on what many perceive as deprivation. I feel this will reinforce positive behaviors, whether or not weight loss is actually achieved.

Let's face it, most children are active to some extent, but the point is to make it a regimented activity so it becomes second nature that there is time for exercise, just like there is time for school and time for play, built into each day. Starting with 5 minutes, I then have my patients increase the time by 5 minutes each day every two weeks until they have gotten to 30 to 45 minutes of exercise. This may seem like a slow process, but bear with it and do not accelerate beyond this rate. It may take several months to build up to a large level of exercise, but that doesn't matter. If you think "lifelong nutritional plan," as you should, then suddenly a few months is meaningless.

This gradual pace serves two purposes. The first is a gradual buildup of time that even the most out-of-shape child can manage, hence eliminating any reason to fail. The second is to ensure that this level of activity increases so gradually that the increase in time becomes unnoticeable. Again, this eliminates the failure rate, and it works quite well for my young patients. All too often, patients will embark on an exercise regime, thinking they can train their child like an Olympic athlete. Not only will this set your child up for failure, but he or she may injure themselves in the process. We are looking for success and results — and remember, they don't have to occur overnight.

some advice for athletes

There is always some possibility of exercise-related injuries, but most can be avoided if you follow some simple rules:

❖ *Force fluids.* Dehydration occurs very frequently, especially in the warmer weather. Too little water can lead to muscle aches, fatigue and even fainting. Your child should drink water before beginning any exercise and then drink 3 ounces of water for every 15 minutes of exercise.

❖ *Warm up.* This should include some minor stretching routines designed specifically to stretch the muscles that are going to be involved in the sport your child is playing. Warming up should help to avoid overuse injuries. These injuries arise when your child is participating in too vigorous a workout.

❖ *If your child experiences pain from a workout, stop the exercise immediately and get to a doctor.* Depending on the injury, your active child may still be able to participate in a different sport, one that does not put much emphasis on the muscle or the bone that is presently injured. For example, a runner suffering from a stress fracture will usually be able to swim until the stress fracture heals.

❖ *Watch out for steroid use.* This is a particularly worrisome problem in the adolescent male population. However, a recent study, published in *The Archives of Pediatric and Adolescent Medicine* indicated that as many as 175,000 high school girls took steroids, using them either to become leaner or to build more muscle. In this same study, the figure for boys was twice as high. Be on the lookout for warning signs such as behavioral changes, significant worsening of an acne problem, or a puffy face. Know that some of the long-term side effects of anabolic steroid use are psychological changes; gynecomastia (breast development), impotence, and testicular atrophy in boys; and shrinkage of the breasts, deepening of the voice, and menstrual irregularities in girls.

starting with preschoolers

There is no reason that an exercise program can't start when your child is a toddler. Although this book is not meant for that age group, the fact is that by the time your child reaches preschool age, the bad, sedentary habits may already have taken hold. So why not start early? And if you make exercise fun, there's no reason why your child won't continue some form of exercise well into adulthood.

Because a formal exercise program may be too vigorous for a preschooler, I recommend swimming classes. It is never too early to start to learn how to swim. Playing around in the water may burn 150 calories in 20 to 30 minutes, depending on the level of activity; and this is a relatively inexpensive way to spend some play time with your child that you can both enjoy.

Dance classes are another great idea for children of this age. And, with the rise in popularity of gymnastics, this is a great age to start with classes structured to the abilities of a preschooler.

Another activity that I have found to work really well is playing physically active games with friends the same age. Preschoolers are generally imaginative and can think of all sorts of games to play without much thought on your part. They love to run, jump, chase, and tag each other at this age. Soccer is a great sport that involves agility and the combination of many things kids like to do anyway. All they need is a ball that can be kicked around and a small space. If your yard's not big enough, then the park or even the school yard will suffice. In New York City, the school yards were where many of my outdoor activities took place. Concrete works just as well as grass. Your child just needs a venue; this is something that can be provided simply with a little organization on your part and the parts of the parents of your child's friends. Organize play dates on a regular basis with alternating parents taking the responsibility. If you are always at work, try to enroll older siblings or the person who watches your child after school now anyway.

For preschoolers, you may want to increase the level of their daily activities such as walking to a store rather than driving or asking them to help with some of the minor chores around the house, such as making their own bed or taking out the trash. Any increase in physical activity is a step in the right direction.

school-age children

The parents of my school-age children never fail to astonish me with their reply to my request for their children to get some form of regimented exercise. "There's not enough time," they say, and I often can't help but wonder which one does not have enough time, the parent or the child? The sad stories I get include excuses like, "My child has homework, after school activities, maybe a music or some other type of lesson — where will they ever find the time to exercise?"

Examine your child's time more closely. Is there time spent talking to friends on the telephone? Is there time in between one of these many activities? Is there time for television? Is there time to be in front of a computer surfing the web? If the answer is yes to any of these questions — and I know it will be — then there is time for exercise. I'm not saying there should not be time in a child's day for simply doing what he or she wishes and for having fun. But what about making exercise fun? That's what it's all about. We want your child to opt for exercise rather than for sitting in front of the television set. But we have to make lifestyle adjustments as early as possible to accomplish this goal.

"I'm too tired"

Children of this age should never be allowed to use the excuse that they are too tired. A child cannot be too tired unless he or she has a physical illness. Children are less often tired than they are unmotivated. Sedentary habits are difficult to break, and if they are a normal American child, these habits have been forming since birth.

The one thing about exercise that always needs a little explanation is this: An exercise program will initially fatigue your child. This occurs because the muscles and lungs are doing things that they are not used to doing. After a period of days to weeks, depending on the level of exercise, your child's muscles will become better trained and more energized. If you think back to how exercise works, your child's muscles will now be more efficient, and this leads to a heightened sense of well-being and much less fatigue.

Parents must provide the motivation for this change in their child by setting the right example. This should be easy because more adults are physically active than their children today. While children become more sedentary, adults are in the midst of a continuing fitness boom that shows little sign of abating. Exercising with your child will inevitably bring you closer together.

I know this may sound impossible, but I urge parents to look at their own lives to see where the downtime is so that exercise can be fit in. Often, though, a parent's downtime and the child's downtime may not overlap. If that's the case, it is still your responsibility as a parent to ensure that your child is getting adequate exercise.

If your child is interested, involve them in organized sporting activities, but don't force them. This will only make your child hate them more. I speak from experience on this one because my parents forced me to play basketball and football, which I was not good at and grew to hate because they were imposed on me against my will.

It has taken me many years to finally get over my hatred of these two sports. It is only in the past few years that I have come to enjoy them and may at times even watch them on television.

household chores

Don't underestimate the power of household chores. They are necessary in every home, and in your busy day, if your children can help you, it will help them as well. Chores such as vacuuming or walking the dog can be great forms of exercise. Buy an active pet such as a dog. Think of all the energy your child can burn just by running and playing with an overactive puppy.

golf

Golf is a great sport for kids to learn because it is a sport in which you are essentially playing against yourself. That was the primary reason why I took up this sport and why I continue to enjoy it. Besides, it's great exercise if you walk the course and a round lasts for several hours. Because of the game's increasing popularity and the demand for equipment and tee times, this can only help make the game more affordable for everyone. It is no longer the rich man's sport that it was when I was a kid. Even if your child is too young to play, but you do, designate a time to bring him or her along. Not only will they learn to appreciate the game, but they will benefit from the exercise of walking, especially if you're playing a hilly course.

use video as an ally

Another effective tool I have found is to use the home exercise tapes featuring famous people whom your children may admire and be comfortable with. Do the exercise tape with them. The level of activity may be too intense for some of the younger kids, but they will do as much as they can.

I often get inspiration from my patients and their families. I had one little girl who used to love doing exercise tapes with her mother. The tape her mother preferred was the Jane Fonda aerobic workout. Today, this might be a little outdated, but it still works. Other, more popular tapes may be ones from The Firm and The Grind, which incorporate more up-to-date music and steps. This particular young patient's mother even made little weights out of canned goods and got her daughter her own little exercise mat. They made the workout resemble the tape as closely as they could. The little girl loved it and would often insist that they do this workout every day. It was now the daughter encouraging the mother to exercise. It does not matter from where the inspiration comes, but it's great when it can be transferred to the child. It became so enjoyable, almost like a game for the child, and she loved it.

adolescence

If your child has made it to adolescence and is still a couch potato, then you have your work cut out for you. It will not be an impossible task, but certainly it will be more difficult than if those sedentary habits had been broken in the younger, more formative years.

To make matters worse, these teenage years are also the ones when kids don't want to take advice from their parents, the enemy. At this age, it is also impossible to oversee everything your child is doing. So, all you can really do is offer guidance and encouragement.

What you can do is make it as easy as possible for them to be successful. Remove any obstacles that could possibly deter them. For example, get them a gym membership or some gym equipment; take away their ability to use the car for simple errands; make them take on more responsibility for cleaning the house or for yard work.

The same suggestions essentially apply to all the age groups. There are competitive sports and individual sports, as well as individual training for adolescents. As far as this goes, for both boys and girls, weight training coupled with aerobic activity is essential. The days of thinking of aerobic activity as the be all and end all of physical fitness has drawn to a close. Each generation has a set of experiences that are uniquely their own. My generation had the aerobics and disco craze. We now believe that in order to maintain a proper workout, aerobic activity must be coupled with weight training, and that's what I'm asking you to encourage in your children.

Weight training is essential for any overweight teenager because it may shift the body metabolism into high gear — possibly for several hours after the exercise has been completed. One study showed that the metabolic rate of people who lifted weights was 7.5 percent higher for 15 hours after they worked out. This is a great advantage for anyone who wants to lose weight, not just children. For most overweight kids, they not only eat more than their normal-weight peers, but expend less energy. If they are encouraged to start a weight-lifting program, they can boost their metabolism and burn more energy more efficiently.

A beginner should probably lift two to three times per week, using weights that can allow eight to twelve repetitions but not much more than that. You can then switch to a heavier weight only after this becomes too easy at the original weight.

A proper exercise regime for an adolescent should include aerobic activity. This can include running, fast walking, biking, or hiking. With my patients, I recommend starting 15 or 20 minutes three times per week, gradually increasing the intensity up to 45 minutes per session and then increasing the days to four or five at the maximum.

Adolescents should be encouraged to participate in organized sports offered in school or at the local level if they are so inclined. Don't force your children to participate in anything they don't want to do. Gentle encouragement is always the key to any successful exercise program.

PART FIVE

Meal Plans

and

Recipes

Sample Menu
Selections

As you will see, the two weeks' worth of menus that follow can be used on Phase 1 of the diet for all age groups. I've tried to make these menus as broadly based as I could so they would apply to the parents of all the children who need this book. When serving your children, keep in mind what I've discussed about portion control. Any child, but especially those who are overweight, must learn this as part of an overall healthy eating plan.

Please exercise good judgment when using these menus. Make the appropriate substitutions as needed for your child. Also keep in mind that foods may be repeated, if desired, as long as you are following the previously outlined rules. Lunch items will vary depending upon where your child will be eating lunch: school, home, or some variation or combination of the two. Use your imagination. And remember, if your child prefers the same thing over and over, you may allow it —as long as it's on the nutritional lifestyle plan I've just outlined.

The numbers in parentheses are the number of grams of carbohydrates for one serving of each meal selection.

go organic

One other thing to keep in mind when reading this section or when preparing these foods is that I prefer that you use organically grown or organically raised food whenever possible. This includes all the vegetables, meats, eggs, cheeses, and so on. As I've explained before, you don't have to eat organically to remain on this diet, but for health reasons, it's important to remember that if you have a choice, go organic.

Another thing to consider is the issue of nitrates and nitrites. These substances, found in cured meats such as lunch meats and bacon, are potentially hazardous to your child's health, and I discourage their use. It has been postulated that these preservatives become nitrosamines in the digestive tract, where they may be implicated in cancer. But, like my caveat about organic foods, nitrate- and nitrite-free versions are available, and in any case, your child can still eat bacon and lunch meats while remaining on the diet. It is just healthier not to.

Have fun with this, and remember that this is only a sampling of the many delicious options you can create for the entire family with the foods available. Recipes for most of the following dishes can be found in the next chapter. I'm allowing you to use some of your family's favorite dishes as well, such as rib eye steak or roast chicken or tuna salad with a couple of restrictions, which are given in the meal plans.

The menu plan below indicates one serving size of the recipes in Chapter 31.

Week 1

Monday

Total grams of carbohydrates for Monday: 39.2

BREAKFAST: Pancakes with 1 serving Strawberry Puree Topping (7.9)
8 ounces Chocolatey Soy Milk (4.0)

In my clinical experience, I've found unsweetened soy milk to be better tolerated by even the most milk-sensitive of patients. The protein structure of the milk is less allergenic, and I feel that it is a healthier product because it has almost no sugar in it.

LUNCH: Cheeseburger (See Variation of recipe for Basic Burger) served on a bed of iceberg lettuce (2.5)
2 Peanut Butter Cookies (3.6)
Fruit-flavored seltzer (0)

As I mentioned in the diet chapters, the cheese on the burger can be any type your child prefers, except for processed American cheese, which is really not cheese at all but rather a food product.

DINNER: Country Chicken (12.2)
1 cup salad with permitted salad dressing (2.0)
Whipped Cauliflower (6.0)
Diet gelatin with a dollop of whipped cream (1.0)
Flavored seltzer

Tuesday

Total grams of carbohydrates for Tuesday: 31.9

BREAKFAST: 2 Basic Scrambled Eggs (0)
8 ounces Chocolatey Soy Milk (4.0)

LUNCH: Tuna salad (1 can tuna packed in water with mayonnaise to taste) on a bed of lettuce (0)

2 Chocolate Almond Cookies (3.9)

Fruit-flavored seltzer (0)

DINNER: Oriental Beef Kebobs (3.6)

¼ cup long grain steamed brown rice (13.0)

1 cup loosely packed lettuce with 1 serving permitted salad dressing (2.0)

1 Mini Sour Cream Cheesecake with 1 serving Strawberry Puree Topping (5.4)

Flavored seltzer (0)

Wednesday

Total grams of carbohydrates for Wednesday: 31.9

BREAKFAST: Pancakes with 1 serving Strawberry Puree Topping (7.9)

1 slice Canadian bacon (nitrate-free, if possible) (0)

8 ounces plain unsweetened soy milk (4.0)

It's difficult but not impossible to buy nitrate-free Canadian bacon. It's worth the time to shop around.

LUNCH: Chicken salad (cold diced chicken with mayonnaise to taste) on a bed of lettuce, season to taste (2)

Fudgie Brownie Square (4.4)

Flavored seltzer (0)

DINNER: My Mother's Meatloaf (3.1)

1 cup salad with permitted salad dressing (2.0)

Baked cauliflower with cheese (variation of broccoli and cheese recipe) (6.0)

1 Mini Sour Cream Cheesecake (2.5)

Flavored seltzer (0)

Thursday

Total grams of carbohydrates for Thursday: 30.0

BREAKFAST: ½ cup puffed kamut cereal with 4 ounces
unsweetened soy milk (7.5)

LUNCH: 1 or 2 turkey hot dogs (0)
Diet gelatin with dollop of whipped cream (1.0)
Flavored seltzer (0)

DINNER: Grilled Pork Oriental (2.0)
1 cup salad with permitted salad dressing (2.0)
½ cup steamed zucchini (3.5)
¼ cup long grain steamed brown rice (13.0)
Diet gelatin with a dollop of whipped cream (1.0)
Flavored seltzer (0)

Friday

Total grams of carbohydrates for Friday: 32.6

BREAKFAST: Basic Omelet (0)
2 turkey sausage links (0)
8 ounces Strawberry Soy Milk (See *Variation* of
recipe for Chocolatey Soy Milk) (5.0)

LUNCH: Turkey Burgers Stuffed with Salsa and Mozzarella (11.0)
Diet gelatin with a dollop of whipped cream (1.0)
Flavored seltzer (0)

DINNER: 2 Hamptons-style Cod Fish Cakes (6.2)
1 cup salad with permitted salad dressing (2.0)
½ cup steamed spinach (3.4)
4 ounces strawberry sorbet (4.0)
Flavored seltzer (0)

Saturday

Total grams of carbohydrates for Saturday: 33.4 or 34.9

BREAKFAST: Basic Omelet with cheese (2.0)
8 ounces Chocolatey Soy Milk (4.0)

LUNCH: 1 or 2 Texas Tommy's (1.5 or 3.0)
2 Chocolate Almond Cookies (3.9)
Seltzer (0)

DINNER: Mary's Village-style Spare Ribs (0)
¼ cup long grain steamed brown rice (13.0)
1 cup salad with permitted salad dressing (2.0)
4 spears steamed asparagus (2.6)
Fudgy Brownie Square (4.4)
Seltzer (0)

Sunday

Total grams of carbohydrates for Sunday: 35.6

BREAKFAST: ½ cup puffed kamut cereal with 4 ounces unsweetened soy milk (7.5)

LUNCH: Steve's Texas Tacos (2.3)
Fudgy Brownie Square (4.4)
Seltzer (0)

DINNER: Chicken Fingers with Sweet Mustard Dipping Sauce (5.4)
1 cup salad with permitted salad dressing (2.0)
Broccoli and Cheese Casserole (8.0)
4 ounces Creamy Cantaloupe Frozen Dessert (6.0)
Seltzer or water (0)

Week 2

Monday

Total grams of carbohydrates for Monday: 35.2

BREAKFAST: Pancakes with butter and 1 serving of Strawberry
Puree Topping (7.9)

8 ounces Chocolatey Soy Milk (4.0)

LUNCH: Grilled Chicken Breast, no sauce (sauté one chicken
breast in olive oil) with 2 tablespoons of grilled
onions (2.0)

Broccoli and Cheese Casserole (8.0)

Flavored seltzer (0)

DINNER: 8-10 ounce broiled rib eye steak, no sauce; season
to taste (0)

Large three-leaf lettuce salad with permitted salad
dressing (2.0)

String Bean and Cheese Casserole (See *Variation*
of recipe for Broccoli and Cheese Casserole) (6.0)

4 ounces of Creamy Strawberry Frozen Dessert (5.3)

Water (0)

Tuesday

Total grams of carbohydrates for Tuesday: 36.9

BREAKFAST: Basic Omelet with spinach and feta cheese (3.0)

8 ounces Strawberry Soy Milk (See *Variation* of recipe
for Chocolatey Soy Milk) (5.0)

LUNCH: Beef Stir-Fry with vegetables (4.3)

           ¼ cup brown rice (13.0)

           Diet gelatin (0)

           Water (0)

DINNER: Roast turkey (any way your family likes it, but no stuffing or sauce allowed) (0)

           Large green salad with permitted salad dressing (2.0)

           Whipped cauliflower and broccoli (See *Variation* of recipe for Whipped Cauliflower) (6.0)

           2 Peanut Butter Cookies (3.6)

           Flavored seltzer (0)

Wednesday

Total grams of carbohydrates for Wednesday : 37.5

BREAKFAST: ½ cup puffed kamut cereal with 4 ounces unsweetened soy milk (7.5)

LUNCH: Egg salad (chopped boiled eggs, mixed with mayonnaise to taste); season to taste (0)

           Salad with permitted salad dressing (2.0)

           2 Chocolate Almond Cookies (3.9)

           Seltzer (0)

DINNER: Veal Parmesan (See *Variation* of recipe for Chicken Fingers) (7.1)

           Roasted Acorn Squash (1/2 cup) (14.0)

           Large green salad with permitted salad dressing (2.0)

           Diet gelatin with a dollop of whipped cream (1.0)

           Water (0)

Thursday

Total grams of carbohydrates for Thursday: 36.9

BREAKFAST: 2 poached eggs (2.0)
1 slice of Canadian bacon (preferably nitrate-free) (0)
8 ounces Chocolatey Soy Milk (4.0)

LUNCH: Tuna salad with mayonnaise (tuna packed in water, mixed with mayonnaise to taste), garnished with chopped celery (1.0)
Fudgy Brownie Square (4.4)
Water (0)

DINNER: Chicken Chunks with Broccoli in a Cheesey Cream Dill Sauce (See *Variation* for Broccoli and Cheese) (8.0)
¼ cup of brown rice (13.0)
Large green salad with permitted salad dressing (2.0)
Mini Sour Cream Cheesecake (2.5)
Flavored seltzer (0)

Friday

Total grams of carbohydrates for Friday: 39.9

BREAKFAST: Cold chicken slices with ¼ cup cottage cheese (4.0)
8 ounces Strawberry Soy Milk (See *Variation* of recipe for Chocolatey Soy Milk) (5.0)

LUNCH: Cheddar Cheeseburger garnished with sautéed
           onions on a bed of lettuce (See *Variation* of
           recipe for Basic Burger) (4.5)
           Fudgy Brownie Square (4.4)
           Flavored seltzer (0)

DINNER: Roast chicken (any way your family likes it, but no
           stuffing or sauce allowed) (0)
           ½ sweet potato with butter (13.0)
           Large green salad with permitted salad dressing (2.0)
           Spinach and Cheese Casserole (See *Variation* of recipe
           for Broccoli and Cheese Casserole) (6.0)
           Diet gelatin with a dollop of whipped cream (1.0)
           Water (0)

Saturday

Total grams of carbohydrates for Saturday: 28.0

BREAKFAST: Basic Omelet with hot dog (2.0)
            8 ounces Strawberry Soy Milk (See *Variation* of recipe
            for Chocolatey Soy Milk) (5.0)

LUNCH: Chicken salad (chicken from Friday's dinner, mixed
            with mayonnaise to taste), garnished with chopped
            celery on a bed of lettuce (1.0)
            Fudgy Brownie Square (4.4)
            Water (0)

DINNER: Chicken Chili (See *Variation* of recipe for Steve's
            Texas Tacos) (2.3)
            Large green salad with permitted salad dressing (2.0)
            Whipped Cauliflower (6.0)
            4 ounces Creamy Watermelon Frozen Dessert (5.3)
            Flavored seltzer (0)

Sunday

Total grams of carbohydrates for Sunday: 33.6 or 35.1

BREAKFAST: ½ cup puffed kamut cereal with 4 ounces unsweetened soy milk (7.5)

LUNCH: 1 or 2 Texas Tommy's (1.5 or 3.0)
Green salad with permitted salad dressing (2.0)
2 Peanut Butter Cookies (3.6)
Flavored seltzer (0)

DINNER: Chicken Meatball Soup (2.0)
¼ cup of brown rice (13.0)
Mini Sour Cream Cheesecake with 1 serving of Strawberry Puree Topping (4.0)
Water (0)

As you can see from this menu plan, it was devised with the most stringent child—the teenager—in mind. The amount of carbohydrates falls into the Phase 1 category for the teenager. It, therefore, can be used by any of the children on the Phase 1 diet. Remember, you can serve your child fewer carbohydrates than I've specified, but not more than I've recommended. In any case, never serve your child fewer than 30 grams of carbohydrates a day.

In order to expand this menu for the two younger categories of children, I recommend adding more salads and vegetables, until you've reached your child's total carbohydrate level as mentioned in the age-specific chapters. It is really quite easy because all we're doing is adding or subtracting grams of carbohydrates as necessary for the different age child. You may refer to one of the many carbohydrate gram counters available in your local bookstores and sit down with your child and plan your own menus.

Now remember, your child will not like everything offered here, nor will he or she need to eat everything that is presented on this menu plan. I offer this only as a general guideline. Make adjustments as necessary, and I encourage you to improvise according to your child's likes and dislikes. If your child likes a particular food, it can be repeated multiple times throughout the week. Don't bully your child into eating anything on the menu plan I've provided simply because it is there. Your child knows what he or she likes, and as long as the food is allowable according to the guidelines I've set up, let them have it as often as they want.

We're asking our children to change their entire way of eating. It is not imperative that they learn to like new foods, at least not in the initial weight-loss phase of the diet. That will come with time. Keep in mind that a diet does not have to be rushed. Children have many years of eating this way ahead of them, and there will be ample time for new foods.

The only hard-and-fast rule that cannot be ignored when you deviate from this menu is that you must watch carbohydrate counts.

In my practice, I've found that my inspiration often comes from the patients themselves. Use your imagination, and allow your children to use theirs. If you come up with something really good, please write and tell me some great recipes you've discovered. I may include them in my next book!

Recipes

I HAD GREAT FUN AND MANY ADVENTURES CREATING THESE RECIPES. You and your family should do the same. There are certain things to keep in mind when preparing recipes. You should almost never use anything labeled "low-fat." As I've said before, once the fat is removed in the processing, something else is generally added, and it is usually sugar —the one substance we are most trying to avoid. You should also try to avoid anything labeled "diet." Again, these products have been processed and usually follow the rules of the common high-carbohydrate dietary regimen. They would most likely not be suitable for this nutritional lifestyle plan.

In the preparation of the desserts, I have included the amounts for liquid saccharin as well as for stevia. In the actual trials of these recipes, I made the desserts in three ways: one with stevia only; the second with a combination of stevia and the liquid saccharin, which I think works the best; and the third way was with the liquid saccharin alone. In the creation of desserts, stevia and liquid saccharin tended to potentiate the sweetening effects of either one alone, allowing me to use less of both, an ideal situation. I report the recipes mostly with liquid saccharin because I feel liquid saccharin is the easiest of the two sweeteners to obtain and I did not want to make these recipes too difficult to follow. It is also the easier of the two to get the proper amount. Under normal circumstances, I'm against the use of artificial sweeteners; however the amount I use is quite low, and I hope that your child will not be eating these all the time. Stevia is a more difficult product to work with and has a much more variable taste because it is more potent than any artificial sweetener. For those who want to try stevia, I have included the amount in each dessert recipe. Please refer to the chapter on sugar, Chapter 4, for more information about stevia.

I should also mention a word about the use of diet gelatin. There are commercial brands on the market that are acceptable to use; however, they contain aspartame, which I feel is not a healthy product for children to be eating. Nevertheless, commercial brands are easier to use, and they can even be bought prepackaged so they fit right in a kid's lunch box. They are therefore permissible; it is just healthier to make your own.

Wherever seltzer is mentioned, it can be flavored or plain, depending on your child's preference. Just make sure it is not flavored with real fruit juice because that will increase the amount of sugar in your child's diet. Seltzer can also be replaced with tap water (filtered, preferably). Because of the phosphorus in carbonated beverages, limit the amount of seltzer your child drinks to 16 ounces a day.

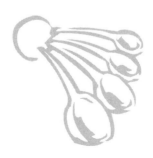

❖ Pancakes ❖

Makes 14 pancakes.
Serving size = 4 pancakes
Total carbohydrates: 19.0
Carbohydrates per serving: 5.4

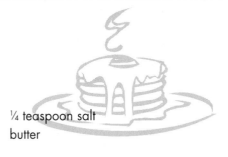

½ cup soy flour
3 eggs
½ cup of water

¼ teaspoon salt
butter

Combine the first four ingredients in a mixing bowl using a hand-held mixer or a wire whisk. Place butter in heated skillet. Allow butter to become piping hot without burning. When this has happened, pour about 1 tablespoon of the batter into the frying pan, allowing time on both sides. Remove the first batch, and continue pouring the batter until all is used.

❖ Strawberry Puree Topping ❖

Makes ⅔ cup puree.
Serving size = ¼ cup puree
Total carbohydrates: 8.0
Carbohydrates per serving: 2.5

This makes a wonderful alternative to syrup. Even the sugar-free syrups are loaded with chemicals. This recipe makes enough to add to unsweetened soy milk and to top off the cheesecake muffins.

5 diced strawberries (average size)

Place the diced strawberries in a food processor or blender. Puree until smooth.

❖ Basic Omelet ❖

Makes 1 omelet.
Serving size = 1 omelet
Total carbohydrates: <2.0
Carbohydrates per serving: <2.0

2 eggs	1½ tablespoons cream (optional)
pinch of pepper	1 to 2 tablespoons butter

Combine first three ingredients in a bowl and beat with a fork until well blended. Melt butter in a skillet, and add the egg mixture. Cook omelet over low heat. To ensure even cooking, lift the edges with a fork or spatula, and tilt pan so raw egg runs underneath. When omelet looks evenly done, fold it in half and serve.

VARIATIONS:

Before folding omelet over, you may add a number of ingredients allowable on the diet that your child will love.

❖ Add 2 ounces shredded cheddar or Swiss cheese, and let melt.

❖ Add 2 tablespoons crumpled fried bacon or Canadian bacon. (You may also add the bacon and the cheese together.)

❖ Add 2 tablespoons sour cream (2 grams of carbohydrates) and a sprinkle of chives.

❖ Add 1 tablespoon sautéed onions (2 grams of carbohydrates) and 2 tablespoons sautéed mushrooms, (2 grams of carbohydrates) or any combination thereof.

❖ Add 1 chopped hot dog.

❖ Add 2 ounces spinach (2 grams of carbohydrates).

❖ Add 1 ounce feta cheese.

❖ Basic Scrambled Eggs ❖

Makes 2 servings.
Serving size = 1 ½ eggs
Total carbohydrates: 2.0
Carbohydrates per serving: 1.0

3 eggs	2 tablespoons cream (optional)
pinch of salt	1 to 2 tablespoons butter
pinch of pepper	

Combine first four ingredients in a bowl and beat with a fork until well blended. Melt butter in a skillet, and add the egg mixture. As you cook eggs over low heat, stir through eggs with a wooden spoon until they become soft, creamy curds.

VARIATIONS:

About one minute before the eggs are done, add one of the following:

- ❖ 2 ounces shredded cheddar or Swiss cheese
- ❖ 2 tablespoons sour cream (2 grams carbohydrates) and a sprinkle of chives
- ❖ Crisp bacon bits (homemade)
- ❖ 2 tablespoons of chopped sautéed onions (2 grams carbohydrates)
- ❖ ¼ cup sautéed mushrooms (2 grams carbohydrates)
- ❖ Bits of broiled sausage (1 gram carbohydrates)

Chocolatey Soy Milk ❖

Makes 1 serving.
Serving size = 1 glass
Total carbohydrates: 4.0
Carbohydrates per serving: 4.0

> 8 ounces unsweetened soy milk
> ½ teaspoon Chocolate No-Cal syrup

Combine ingredients in a glass, and stir until well mixed.

VARIATION:

❖ Strawberry Soy Milk—Add ¼ teaspoon Strawberry Puree Topping in place of chocolate syrup (see page 257). Carbohydrates per serving: 5.0.

❖ Basic Burger ❖

Makes 4 servings.
Serving size = 1 burger
Total carbohydrates: 2.0
Carbohydrates per serving: 0.5

> 1½ pounds ground beef   ¼ teaspoon pepper
>   or ground turkey   1 egg
> ¼ cup chopped parsley   1 tablespoon tomato paste (optional)
> ¼ cup chopped onion
> ½ teaspoon salt

Mix all ingredients in a bowl and divide into 4 burgers. Grill under broiler or in a skillet until burger is cooked to suit your child's taste. In order to avoid contamination, it is best to cook all meat well through or until meat thermometer gets to 160 degrees.

VARIATIONS:

❖ Cheeseburger: Top burger with 2 ounces of ch‹ Swiss cheese, or other allowable cheese your cl ‹‹‹‹‹ ‹‹‹‹. Carbohydrates per serving: 2.5

❖ Pizza Burger: Top burger with ½ tablespoon tomato paste and 2 ounces shredded whole-milk mozzarella. Carbohydrates per serving: 3.5

❖ Bacon Burger: Top burger with one or two strips of crisp nitrate-free bacon. Carbohydrates per serving: 0.5

❖ Bacon Cheeseburger: Top burger with one or two strips of crisp nitrate-free bacon and 2 ounces cheddar or other acceptable cheese. Carbohydrates per serving: 2.5

❖ Veggie Burger: Top burger with 2 tablespoons chopped sautéed onions, mushrooms, or green pepper. 1 ounce cheese goes well on top of this. Grams of carbohydrates for this variation depend on the ingredients chosen—2 tablespoons onions: 3.5; 2 tablespoons mushrooms: 2.5; 2 tablespoons green pepper: 2.1; cheese: 2.

❖ Beef Stir-Fry ❖

Makes 4 servings.
Serving size = 1 bowl
Total carbohydrates: 17.2
Carbohydrates per serving: 4.3

1 tablespoon olive oil
4 ounces onions, diced
1 pound beef, thinly sliced

4 ounces broccoli, chopped
4 ounces cauliflower, chopped
4 ounces green beans, sliced

Sauté onions in olive oil until slightly brown, then add meat. When meat is almost cooked, add a small amount of water and the vegetables. Cover for 1 minute. Remove cover and continue cooking for 5 more minutes. Do not overcook the vegetables.

❖ Texas Tommy's ❖

Makes 2 servings.
Serving size = 1 hot dog
Total carbohydrates: 3.0
Carbohydrates per serving: 1.5

2 beef hot dogs (without
  nitrates if possible)

1 tablespoon butter
3 ounces cheddar cheese

Melt butter in a skillet. Place hot dogs on skillet, and grill hot dogs until they are heated through.

Remove them from skillet and split them about halfway down along the length of the hot dog. Push cheese into the splits and place in 350 degree oven for a few minutes, or until cheese is melted.

❖ Steve's Texas Tacos ❖

Makes 6 servings.
Serving size = 2 tacos
Total carbohydrates: 14.0
Carbohydrates per serving: 2.3

1 pound ground beef
¼ cup chopped onion
1 tablespoon tomato paste
⅛ teaspoon each thyme,
  cumin, and chili powder
⅛ teaspoon paprika

1 teaspoon salt
pinch cayenne pepper (optional)
crisp fresh lettuce leaves
4 ounces grated jack cheese
4 tablespoons sour cream

Sauté ground beef and onion in a skillet over medium-high heat until the meat is no longer pink. Remove from heat and drain off the liquid. Add tomato paste, thyme, cumin, chili powder, paprika, salt, and cayenne. Continue to sauté until meat is thoroughly cooked. Take 1 to 2 tablespoons of the ground beef and place it toward the edge of one of the lettuce leaves. Sprinkle ½ ounce cheese across the beef. Add 1 teaspoon sour cream. Roll up ingredients in the lettuce leaf and serve.

VARIATIONS:

❖ Chicken, Turkey, or Pork Chili: Use shredded cooked chicken, turkey, or pork to replace the ground beef and serve in a bowl, topped with the cheese and sour cream. Note: Using different meat will not affect the carbohydrate count.

❖ Chicken Meatball Soup ❖

Makes 15 servings.
Serving size = 1 Bowl
Total carbohydrates: 30.0
Carbohydrates per serving: 2.0

96 ounces chicken broth
  (the kind without MSG)
20 ounces water
3 7 ½-inch stalks celery
2 whole chicken breasts, split
1 bunch dill, chopped

½ bunch parsley, chopped
1 cup sliced mushrooms
1 pound ground beef
salt to taste
pepper to taste

Place broth and water in a large pot. Dice celery. Add chicken, dill, parsley, mushrooms, and celery to liquid in pot. Bring to boil, lower heat, and simmer covered for 45 minutes. Remove chicken from soup and let stand until cool enough to handle. Meanwhile, roll the ground meat into bite size balls and place them into soup for 20 minutes. Remove skin from cooled chicken, and pull meat from the bones. Cut chicken into bite size pieces. Replace the chicken into the soup. Simmer additional 10 minutes. Add salt and pepper to taste and enjoy. (If your child prefers a spicier soup, you can add red pepper flakes to taste.)

key Burgers Stuffed with ❖ Salsa and Mozzarella

Makes 3 servings.
Serving size = 2 burgers (for younger children, one burger is sufficient.)
Total carbohydrates: 33.0
Carbohydrates per serving: 11.0

6 ounces finely
chopped tomato
1 tablespoon chopped
red onion
1 small clove garlic, minced
2 tablespoons chopped
fresh cilantro

1 tablespoon chopped fresh parsley
½ cup shredded mozzarella
2 teaspoons olive oil
¾ pound ground white-meat turkey
salt to taste
black pepper to taste

Combine all ingredients into a bowl, and shape into 6 burgers. Cook in the broiler or in a skillet until they are browned on both sides, roughly 6 to 8 minutes.

❖ Chicken Fingers ❖

Makes 5 servings.
Serving size = 6 fingers
Total carbohydrates: 27.0
Carbohydrates per serving: 5.4

2 eggs
2 ounces unsweetened
soy milk
salt to taste
pepper to taste

1¼ pounds sliced, boneless,
skinless chicken breasts
¾ cup soy flour
olive oil

Beat eggs until smooth. Combine eggs with soy milk, salt, and pepper to create an egg wash. Cut the chicken breasts into 30 thin, finger-like strips. Place the soy flour into a large bottomed bowl. After this is done, place enough olive oil in a skillet to coat the bottom of the skillet and then a little more. This oil must get piping hot.

While waiting for the oil to get hot, take the chicken finge
the egg wash, then dip in the bowl with the soy flour, coverir   ......
Place in a dish until all have been coated. By this time, the oil should be
hot enough. Place the coated chicken into the oil and fry on both sides
5 to 6 minutes, or until golden brown. Place these on a dish that has
been lined with paper towels to soak up any of the extra oil. Serve with
dipping sauce. See following two recipes for some suggestions.

VARIATION:

❖ Veal Parmesan: Use veal in place of chicken. When veal fingers
   are browned, drain oil from skillet. Sprinkle veal with shredded
   mozzarella cheese. Cover pan, and cook veal over medium-low
   heat until meat is cooked through and cheese is melted.

❖ Sweet Mustard Dipping Sauce ❖

Makes 1 serving.
Serving size = 1½ tablespoons
Total carbohydrates: 0
Carbohydrates per serving: 0

*This is similar to the honey mustard sauce found at fast food restaurants that
kids just seem to love.*

½ teaspoon olive oil   1 tablespoon Dijon mustard
5 drops liquid stevia or
   10 drops liquid saccharin

Combine all ingredients in a bowl.

❖ Eastern Influence Dipping Sauce ❖

Makes 3 servings.
Serving size = 2 tablespoons
Total carbohydrates: 6.0
Carbohydrates per serving: 2.0

2 tablespoons unsweetened
   soy sauce
1 tablespoon lime juice

2 tablespoons water
1 teaspoon ground ginger
½ teaspoon olive oil

Combine all ingredients in a bowl.

❖ Country Chicken ❖

Makes 6 servings.
Serving size = 1 bowl
Total carbohydrates: 73.2
Carbohydrates per serving: 12.2

3½ pound chicken
1 tablespoon olive oil
1 medium red onion, diced
4 cloves garlic, minced
1 red pepper, diced
1 green pepper, diced
1 teaspoon dried thyme
½ teaspoon dried rosemary

½ teaspoon dried oregano
10 ounces mushrooms, cut in quarters
28-ounce can whole plum tomatoes
1 bay leaf
salt to taste
pepper to taste
6 tablespoons grated parmesan
   cheese

Cut the chicken into pieces, splitting the breast. Remove and discard skin. Heat oil in a large, deep skillet, and add chicken. Brown and turn pieces. Add onion, garlic, red and green peppers, thyme, rosemary, and oregano. Allow the vegetables to soften for 5 minutes. Add mushrooms and cook for another 5 minutes. Add the tomatoes and the bay leaf, and simmer on low heat for 50 minutes. Remove the bay leaf. Add salt and pepper to taste.

Remove the chicken. Allow to cool and then cut meat off the bone in large chunks and toss back into the pot. Reheat. Plate this into large bowls, and top with grated parmesan cheese.

❖ Mary's Village-style Spare

Makes 6 servings.
Serving size = About 4 to 6 ribs
Total carbohydrates: 2.0
Carbohydrates per serving: Negligible

This is one of the many recipes that my patients have shared with me through-out the years, and the woman who gave me this personal favorite is one of the best cooks I've ever met.

2 pounds spare ribs
(beef or pork,
whichever your
child prefers)
2 tablespoons sugar-free
soy sauce
1 teaspoon cayenne, or chili
powder, or a combination
of the two

1 tablespoon dried thyme
2 tablespoons dried rosemary
15 drops liquid stevia or 30
drops liquid saccharin
1 teaspoon salt
1 clove garlic, grated
3 tablespoons olive oil

Put ribs in a roasting pan. Combine all the other ingredients in a bowl and mix thoroughly. Pour over the ribs, and rub them so all sides are coated with the mixture. Place in a 375 degree oven, basting the ribs every 15 minutes. If the sauce runs dry, add some water to the bottom of the pan and continue to baste. Bake for about 1 hour, or until crispy on the outside. Serve with the delicious dipping sauce that follows.

❖ Ribs Dipping Sauce ❖

Makes 6 servings.
Serving size = 2 ounces
Total carbohydrates: 6.0
Carbohydrates per serving: 1.0

    1 bunch Italian parsley, finely chopped
    1 bunch mint, finely chopped
    1 bunch curly parsley, finely chopped
    1 tablespoon capers, rinsed and dried
        then finely chopped
    2 hard boiled egg yolks, mashed
    2 cloves garlic, crushed and grated
    ¼ pint olive oil
    salt to taste
    pepper to taste

Place the parsleys and the mint in a food processor and blend. Place in a bowl and set aside. In another bowl, mix the capers and the egg yolks together, and then add to the parsley mixture and blend together. Then add garlic, salt, pepper, and olive oil gradually until the desired taste and consistency is reached.

VARIATION:

❖ Add 2 tablespoons lemon or 2 tablespoons white wine vinegar. Either is delicious.

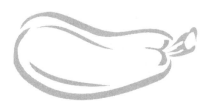

❖ Oriental Beef Kebobs ❖

Makes 8 servings.
Serving size = 1 kebob
Total carbohydrates: 29.0
Carbohydrates per serving: 3.6

¼ cup olive oil
¾ teaspoon black pepper
½ teaspoon cayenne
2 tablespoons low-sodium
   sugar-free soy sauce
2 tablespoons lime juice
¼ teaspoon cumin
1 teaspoon salt
1 tablespoon chopped garlic

2 tablespoons sesame oil
5 pounds lean beef,
   cut into 1-inch cubes
8 wooden skewers
16 medium-size mushroom caps
1 medium green pepper
1 medium red pepper
1 medium onion

In a large bowl, combine olive oil, black pepper, cayenne, soy sauce, lime juice, cumin, salt, garlic, and sesame oil. Add beef cubes. Toss and coat the meat well. Set in the refrigerator covered for at least an hour; overnight is even better. Soak wooden skewers in water.

When ready, peel and clean the mushrooms and set aside. Cut the peppers and onion into bite-size squares. Place all vegetables into a pot of boiling water and parboil for about 2 minutes. Drain these vegetables. Arrange beef and vegetables on the skewers. I usually arrange them: meat cube, onion, green pepper (alternating with red pepper), mushroom cap, and so on. This should be enough to make 8 skewers with 4 cubes of meat on each.

Broil for 8 to 12 minutes, longer if your child prefers meat extra well done. These should be turned and basted periodically with sugar-free soy sauce.

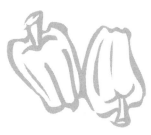

❖ Hamptons-style Cod Fish Cakes ❖

Makes 5 servings.
Serving size = 2 fish cakes
Total carbohydrates: 31.0
Carbohydrates per serving: 6.2

1 pound boneless filleted
   cod, cut into chunks
½ cup diced yam
½ cup chopped onion
2 tablespoons chopped
   fresh parsley

½ teaspoon salt
½ teaspoon pepper
1 egg, well beaten
¼ cup soy flour
olive oil

Put first three ingredients into a pot of boiling water for 7 to 10 minutes until tender. Drain. Put mixture into mixing bowl, and add the parsley, salt, and pepper. Mash all ingredients together, and then add the beaten egg and the soy flour to form a thick batter. If you prefer them a little smoother, then you should mix them together using a blender or food processor.

Heat the olive oil in a skillet until piping hot. Form the batter into 10 fishcakes. Place into the hot oil, and sauté on both sides for about 10 minutes per side or until golden brown. Although these are precooked before they even get to the frying stage, they are best if they are heated thoroughly in the skillet and allowed to turn golden brown on both sides before serving.

❖ My Mother's Meatloaf ❖

Makes 6 servings.
Serving size = 1 slice 1-inch thick
Total carbohydrates: 18.5
Carbohydrates per serving: 3.1

This is a traditional Pescatore family favorite. Although I know my mother would prefer that I keep this recipe in the family, I'm happy to share it with you.

¾ pound each ground veal, pork, and beef	¼ cup diced onion
2 eggs	⅛ teaspoon cumin
3 tablespoons grated Parmesan cheese	¼ teaspoon salt
1 tablespoon chopped garlic	½ teaspoon black pepper
¼ cup fresh chopped parsley	¼ cup unprocessed miller's bran
	2 tablespoons tomato paste
	4 ounces mozzarella cheese, shredded

Combine all ingredients, except tomato paste and mozzarella, in a mixing bowl, using your hands to knead all ingredients together thoroughly. Turn into roasting pan, and form into a loaf 6 to 7 inches long. Place in preheated oven at 375 degrees for 1 hour and 45 minutes.

Remove from oven, and coat top of the loaf with the tomato paste. Then slice into the top of the loaf (about ½ inch deep) horizontally and vertically. Place the shredded cheese in the cuts. Place back in the oven for another 15 minutes.

❖ Grilled Pork Oriental ❖

Makes 3 servings.
Serving size = 4 ounces (3 chunks)
Total carbohydrates: 6.0
Carbohydrates per serving: 2.0

12 ounces pork tenderloin	½ cup dry red wine
1 large clove garlic, minced	1 tablespoon reduced-sodium sugar-free soy sauce
	1 teaspoon Dijon mustard

Trim excess fat from the tenderloin. Cut into 9 chunks and place in glass bowl. In a small saucepan, combine the garlic with the wine, soy sauce, and mustard. Boil this mixture for 2 minutes to thicken. Add to the pork, covering it well. Broil for 8 to 12 minutes, basting with the marinade frequently. Make sure marinade has been cooked sufficiently.

❖ Broccoli and Cheese Casserole ❖

Makes 8 servings.
Serving size = ½ cup
Total carbohydrates: 64.0
Carbohydrates per serving: 8.0

4 cups cooked broccoli flowerets	1 cup unsweetened soy milk
2 tablespoons butter	8 ounces cheddar cheese, shredded
2 tablespoons soy flour	½ teaspoon salt
	½ teaspoon pepper

Place the cooked broccoli in a casserole dish. Melt the butter in a saucepan over medium heat. Whisk the soy flour into the butter at least 2 minutes. (Note this takes longer to thicken than a conventional white sauce because there are no glutens in the soy flour.) Then add the soy milk. Continue whisking until the mixture begins to thicken. Add the cheese, salt, and pepper to the saucepan. Continue to whisk this mixture until velvety smooth. Remove from heat and pour over the broccoli. Place in the oven at 350 degrees for 20 minutes.

VARIATIONS:

❖ String Bean and Cheese Casserole: Use 4 cups cooked, cut string beans in place of broccoli. Carbohydrates per serving: 4.0

❖ Spinach and Cheese Casserole: Use 4 cups cooked, well-drained, chopped spinach in place of broccoli. Carbohydrates per serving: 4.0

❖ Chicken Chunks with Broccoli in a Cheesey Cream Dill Sauce: Add 1 pound cooked, cubed skinless chicken breasts and 2–3 strips of lean, preferably nitrate-free bacon, cooked and crumbled. Add dill to taste. Carbohydrates per serving: 8.0

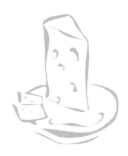

❖ Whipped Cauliflower ❖

Makes 4-6 servings.
Serving size = ¾ cup to 1 cup
Total carbohydrates: 24.0
Carbohydrates per serving: 4.0–6.0 depending on serving size

This can take the place of mashed potatoes.

4 ounces soy milk
3 tablespoons butter
½ teaspoon salt
½ teaspoon pepper
3 strips lean bacon
(preferably nitrate-free)

4 cups cooked cauliflower
2 tablespoons sour cream
4 ounces gruyere cheese, shredded
paprika
3 tablespoons parmesan
cheese, grated

Mash the cauliflower. Then place it in a mixing bowl with the soy milk, butter, sour cream, salt, pepper, and parmesan. With an electric hand mixer, puree all ingredients until there is a thick consistency. Trim the excess fat off 3 strips of bacon, and fry until crisp. Break the bacon into small pieces, and mix through the pureed mixture. Spread into a casserole dish, and top with gruyere. Sprinkle with paprika, if desired. Place in a 350 degree oven for 20 minutes, or until the cheese has melted and the top has browned.

VARIATION:

❖ Whipped Cauliflower and Broccoli: Substitute broccoli for half the cauliflower.

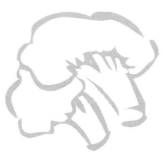

Dressing with Cream Cheese ❖

Serving Size = 2 tablespoons
Total carbohydrates: 6.0
Carbohydrates per serving: 1.0

Any kid will enjoy this and the following Italian dressing.

3 ounces cream cheese
1 teaspoon minced onion
½ teaspoon Dijon mustard
1 teaspoon salt
½ teaspoon black pepper

2 tablespoons chopped
    fresh parsley
¼ cup olive oil
1½ tablespoons white
    wine vinegar

Beat the cream cheese until smooth. Beat in the onion, mustard, salt, pepper, and parsley. Then gradually beat in the olive oil and the vinegar until the desired consistency is reached.

❖ Italian Dressing ❖

Makes 6 servings.
Serving size = 2 tablespoons
Total carbohydrates: 6.0
Carbohydrates per serving: 1.0

⅓ cup white wine vinegar
2 sliced garlic cloves
½ teaspoon dried oregano
¼ teaspoon dried basil

¼ teaspoon dried dill
⅔ cup olive oil
1½ teaspoons lemon juice

Combine the first five ingredients well. Then gradually add the olive oil and the lemon juice until the desired consistency is reached.

VARIATION

For those on a yeast-free diet: Mix only olive oil and fresh-squeezed lemon juice in whatever proportion your child prefers.

❖ Mini Sour Cream Cheesecakes ❖

Makes 12 servings.
Serving size = 1 mini cheesecake
Total carbohydrates: 30.0
Carbohydrates per serving: 2.5

For the crust:
4 tablespoons butter
½ cup miller's bran

20 drops liquid saccharin or
5 drops liquid stevia

Melt the butter in a saucepan. Combine with the miller's bran, and add the sweetener. Take a muffin pan and line with muffin-size baking cups. Put 1 teaspoon of the mixture in the bottom of each cup and press firmly. Place in the refrigerator, and chill for at least one hour. Preheat oven to 375 degrees.

For the cake:
2 well-beaten eggs
1 teaspoon lemon juice
1 tablespoon liquid saccharin
    or 1 teaspoon liquid stevia

¾ pound softened cream cheese
½ teaspoon salt

Mix all ingredients together and beat well with an electric mixer until there is a smooth consistency. Remove the muffin tin from the refrigerator and spoon the batter equally into the cups. Bake for 20 minutes. Remove from the oven and let come to room temperature. In the meantime, preheat the oven to 425 degrees.

For the topping:
¾ cup sour cream
15 drops liquid
    saccharin or 5 drops
    liquid stevia

¼ teaspoon vanilla extract
⅛ teaspoon salt

Mix these ingredients in a small bowl with an electric hand mixer until smooth and creamy. Once the mini cheesecakes have come to room temperature, glaze the tops of each with the sour cream mixture, and place back in the oven for 5 minutes. Remove from the oven and let cool. Refrigerate for 6 to 12 hours before serving.

❖ Fudgy Brownie Squares ❖

Makes 16 servings.
Serving size = 1 square
Total carbohydrates: 70.0
Carbohydrates per serving: 4.4

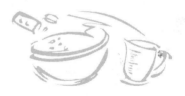

4 ounces unsweetened
    chocolate
1 stick butter
2 tablespoons liquid
    saccharin or 1 teaspoon
    liquid stevia
2 eggs

2 tablespoons water
1½ teaspoons vanilla extract
½ cup soy flour
½ teaspoon baking soda
¼ teaspoon salt
½ cup chopped walnuts

Melt the chocolate in a saucepan over medium heat. Melt the butter with the chocolate. Combine in a mixing bowl the sweetener, eggs, water, and vanilla. Mix vigorously either by hand or with an electric mixer. Add the melted chocolate/butter combination to this mixture and stir well. Next, stir in flour, baking soda, and salt. Then add the nuts, stirring gradually. Spread into a greased 13 x 9-inch baking pan. Bake in preheated 350 degree oven for 15 minutes. Cool in pan. Cut into 16 pieces. They can be cut into smaller pieces depending on the age of your child. (Note: these will not rise like conventional brownies because of the soy flour. They come out more like flat squares, but they taste delicious.)

❖ Chocolate Almond Cookies ❖

Makes 12 servings.
Serving size = 2 cookies
Total carbohydrates: 47.0
Carbohydrates per serving: 3.9

1 ounce unsweetened
    chocolate
2 teaspoons butter

1 cup soy flour
5 teaspoons baking powder
¼ cup water

¼ teaspoon stevia (or forget the saccharin and use
   ¾ teaspoon of stevia only)
40 drops liquid saccharin (or forget the stevia and use
   1 tablespoon of the liquid saccharin only)
1 teaspoon vanilla extract
¼ cup almonds, chopped

Melt the chocolate in a saucepan over medium heat. Melt the butter with the chocolate. Sift together flour and baking powder into a mixing bowl. Then mix together, either by hand or with an electric mixer, the butter, chocolate, water, sweetener(s), and vanilla extract until thoroughly mixed. Add the almonds, and mix through by hand. Drop by teaspoonfuls onto a greased cookie sheet. Place in a preheated 350 degree oven for 12 to 15 minutes. (Note: the cookies taste a lot better than the batter, so don't be alarmed.)

❖ Peanut Butter Cookies ❖

Makes 12 servings.
Serving size = 2 cookies
Total carbohydrates: 44.0
Carbohydrates per serving: 3.6

1 cup soy flour
1½ teaspoons baking
   powder (nonaluminum kind)
2 teaspoons vanilla extract
½ cup water
50 drops liquid saccharin or
   ¼ teaspoon liquid stevia

2 teaspoons butter, melted
4 tablespoons all-natural,
   sugar-free, crunchy peanut
   butter (room temperature)

Combine the flour, baking powder, vanilla extract, water, and sweetener vigorously, either by hand or with an electric mixer. Then add the melted butter and the peanut butter. Combine all ingredients well until a batter is formed. Drop the batter in teaspoon-size lumps onto a greased cookie sheet, and place in a preheated 350 degree oven for 12 to 15 minutes. Allow to cool before serving, although these are great warm, too.

❖ Creamy Strawberry Frozen Dessert ❖

Makes 6 servings.
Serving size = 4 ounces
Total carbohydrates: 32.0
Carbohydrates per serving = 5.3

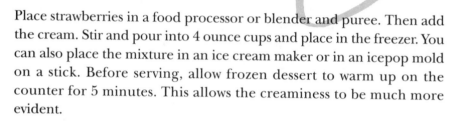

2 cups diced strawberries
¾ cup heavy cream

Place strawberries in a food processor or blender and puree. Then add the cream. Stir and pour into 4 ounce cups and place in the freezer. You can also place the mixture in an ice cream maker or in an icepop mold on a stick. Before serving, allow frozen dessert to warm up on the counter for 5 minutes. This allows the creaminess to be much more evident.

VARIATIONS:

Use pureed cantaloupe or watermelon, which kids really love.

❖ Creamy Cantaloupe Frozen Dessert: Use 2 cups cantaloupe cubes (½-inch) in place of strawberries. Carbohydrates per serving: 6.0

❖ Creamy Watermelon Frozen Dessert: Use 2 cups watermelon cubes (½-inch) in place of strawberries. Carbohydrates per serving: 5.3

References

INTRODUCTION

The statistics on the prevalence of overweight children were taken from: Center for Disease Control, "Third National Health and Nutrition Examination Survey (NHANES III), Update: Prevalence of Overweight among Children, Adolescents, and Adults — United States, 1988 – 1994." *Journal of the American Medical Association*, 277, 14 (April 9, 1997) 199–202.

CHAPTER 2

The reference to a fat-enabling culture was taken from: Kolata, G., "The Fat-Enabling Culture: Society Made Me Eat It!" *New York Times* (December 1, 1996): 4.

The statistics on young girls and dieting were taken from: Waterhouse, Debra, *Like Mother, Like Daughter*. New York: Hyperion, 1997.

CHAPTER 3

The reference to the number of girls who have wanted to diet can be found in: Schrieber, G.B., M. Robins, et al., "Weight Modification Efforts Reported by Black and White Pre-Adolescent Girls. National Heart, Lung, and Blood Institute Growth and Health Study." *Pediatrics* 98 (1996) 63–70.

The reference to the studies on obesity at the cellular level can be found in: Hirsch, J., "Cell Number and Size as a Determinant of Subsequent Obesity." In *Childhood Obesity*, edited by M. Winick: New York, John Wiley & Sons, Inc., 1975.

The studies to which I refer, on the treatment of obesity and published after Hirsch, are:

Stunkard, A. T., Sorenson, et al., "An Adoption Study of Human Obesity." *New England Journal of Medicine*, 314 (1986): 193–198.

Stunkard A. T., Foch T., and Z. Hrubec, "A Twin Study of Human Obesity." *Journal of the American Medical Association*, 256 (1986): 51–54.

Borjeson, M. "The Etiology of Obesity in Children." Acta Paediatrica, 65 (1976): 279–287.

The reference to mother's milk being different from cow's milk can be found in: Weiner, M.A., and K. Goss, *Healing Children Naturally*, San Rafael, CA: Quantum Books, 1993. 31–36.

The reference to the contents of mother's milk can be found in: Levin, B., "Infant Nutrition: Correcting Our Mistakes." *Nutrition Science News* 2, no. 4 (1997): 192.

The reference to carbohydrates as an energy source can be found in: Griffiths, M., et al., "Metabolic Rate and Physical Development in Children at Risk of Obesity." *Lancet* 336 (1990): 76–78.

The reference to low-fat diets for children can be found in: "Lack of Omega-3 Fatty Acids Linked to Childhood Behavioral Problems." *Nutrition Science News* 2, no.4 (1997): 192–194.

CHAPTER 4

The reference to the glycemic index can be found in: Jenkins, D.L. et al., "Glycemic Index of Foods: A Physiologic Basis for Carbohydrate Exchange." *American Journal of Clinical Nutrition* 34 (1981): 362–366.

The figures on the amounts and types of sweeteners and sugars consumed is from: U.S. Department of Agriculture, Economic Research Service, *Sugar and Sweetener Situation and Outlook Report,* 1995.

More information about stevia can be obtained in: Bonvie, L., et al., *The Stevia Story,* Atlanta: B.E.D. Publications, 1997.

CHAPTER 5

The study on extreme fat restriction can be found in: *Journal of the American Medical Association,* "Long-term Cholesterol-lowering Effects of Four Fat-Restricted Diets in Hypercholesterolemic and Combined Hyperlipidemic Men, The Dietary Alternatives Study." Knopp, R.H., C.E. Walden, et al., 278, no. 18 (1997) 1509–1515.

The reference to low-fat diets not being the best idea for children can be found in:
Wilson, C.O. "Low-Fat Foods Stunts Children." *London Sunday Telegraph* (May 12, 1996): 7.

Bar–Or, O. and V.B. Unnithan "Nutritional Requirements of Young Soccer Players." *Journal of Sports Sciences* 12 (1994): 39S–42S.

Additional research on types of fats, fish oils, and pharmacologic effects of lipids can be found in:
Wykes, A.A., ed. *Effects of Fish Oils and Polyunsaturated Omega-3 Fatty Acids in Health and Disease.* Bethesda, MD: National Library of Medicine, National Institutes of Health, 1995.

Siscovick, D.S., et al. "Dietary Intake and Cell Membrane Levels of Long Chain n-e Polyunsaturated Fatty Acids and the Risk of Primary Cardiac Arrest." *Journal of the American Medical Association* 274, no. 17 (1995): 1363–1367.

Willett, W.C., et al. "Intake of Trans Fatty Acids and Risk of Coronary Heart Disease Among Women." *Lancet* 341 (1993): 581–585.

Sardesai, V.M. "The Essential Fatty Acids." *Nutrition in Clinical Practice* 7, no. 4 (1992): 40-43.

Kabara, J.J., ed. "The Pharmacological Effects of Lipids." In meeting journal of *The American Oil Chemists Society,* 1–14. Champaign, IL, 1978.

The reference to oils and cardiac disease prevention can be found in: Alfin-Slater, R.B., and L. Aftergood, *Lipids: Modern Nutrition in Health and Disease,* 6th edition, Chapter 5, 131, edited by R.S. Goodheart and M.E. Shils, Philadelphia, PA: Lea & Febiger, 1980.

The reference concerning heart disease, certain cancers and fatty acids can be found in: Sears, B., "Essential Fatty Acids, Eicosanoids, and Cancer." In *Adjuvant Nutrition in Cancer Treatment,* Chapter 14, edited by P. Quillon and R.S. Williams, Arlington Heights, IL: Cancer Treatment Research Foundation, 1993.

The reference to behavioral problems and essential fatty acids can be found in: Omega-3 Fatty Acids in Nutrition, Vascular Biology, and Medicine: Proceedings from a Scientific Conference, Councils on Arteriosclerosis, Thrombosis, Basic Science and High Blood Pressure Research. The Nutrition Committee and the National Heart, Lung, and Blood Institute. Dallas, TX: The American Heart Association, 1995.

The reference to tropical oils having antimicrobial properties can be found in: Prior, I., et al., "A Study of South Pacific Islanders Who Consumed Large Amounts of Coconut Oil." *American Journal of Nutrition* 34 (1981): 1552.

CHAPTER 6

The reference to sugar being linked to many common disorders can be found in:

Webber, L.S., et al. "Obesity Studies in Bogalusa." *American Journal of Medical Sciences* 310 (1995): 53S–61S.

Gidding, S.S., et al. "Effects of Secular Trends in Obesity on Coronary Risk Factors in Children: The Bogalusa Heart Study." *Journal of Pediatrics* 127 (1995): 868–874.

Pinhas-Hamiel, O., et al. "Non-Insulin Dependent Diabetes Mellitus Is Increasing Among Adolescents." *Pediatric Research* 37 (1995): 7A.

Rocchini, A.P., "Adolescent Obesity and Hypertension." *Pediatric Clinics of North America* 60 (1993): 81–92.

Rocchini, A.P., et al. "Insulin and Renal Sodium Retention in Obese Adolescents." *Hypertension* 14 (1989): 367–374.

The reference to heart disease and sugar consumption can be found in:

Sears, B. "Essential Fatty Acids and Dietary Endocrinology: A Hypothesis for Cardiovascular Treatment." *Journal of Advancement in Medicine* 6, no. 4 (1993), 211–224.

Siguel, E. *Essential Fatty Acids in Health and Disease.* Brookline, MA: Nutrition Press, 1994.

"Omega-3 Fatty Acids in Nutrition, Vascular Biology, and Medicine: Proceedings from a Scientific Conference, Councils on Arteriosclerosis, Thrombosis, Basic Science and High Blood Pressure Research." The Nutrition Committee and the National Heart, Lung, and Blood Institute. Dallas, TX: The American Heart Association, 1995.

CHAPTER 17

The references to the overprescription of antibiotics can be found in:

Wilkoff, W.G. "I'm an Antibiotic Abuser." *Internal Medicine News* (April 15, 1997):13.

McCaig, L.F., and J.M. Hughes "Trends in Antimicrobial Drug Prescribing among Office-Based Physicians in the United States." *Journal of the American Medical Association* 273 (1995): 214–219.

Hamm, R.M., R.J. Hicks and D.A. Demben. "Antibiotics and Respiratory Infections: Are Patients More Satisfied When Expectations Are Met?" *Journal of Family Practice* 43 (1996): 56–62.

Mainous, A.G., 3rd, W.J. Hueston and J.R. Clark. "Antibiotics and Upper Respiratory Infections: Do Some Folks Think There is a Cure for the Common Cold?" *Journal of Family Practice* 42 (1996): 357–361.

CHAPTER 18

The reference to the relationship between decreased insulin levels and lower cholesterol readings can be found in: Nuutinen, O., and M. Knip, "Long-term Weight Control in Obese Children: Persistence of Treatment Outcomes and Metabolic Changes." *International Journal of Obesity and Metabolic Disorders* 16 (1992): 279–287.

The references to insulin, obesity, and chronic illnesses can be found in:

Medalie, J.H., C.M. Papier, et al. "Major Factors in the Development of Diabetes Mellitus in 10,000 Men." *Archives of Internal Medicine* 135 (1975): 811–817.

Mann, G.V. "The Influence of Obesity on Health." *The New England Journal of Medicine* 291 (1974): 178–185 and 226–232.

Barrett-Connor, E.L. "Obesity, Atherosclerosis, and Coronary Artery Disease." *Annals of Internal Medicine* 103 (1985): 1010–1019.

Pi-Sunyer, F.X. "Medical Hazards of Obesity." *Annals of Internal Medicine* 119 (1993): 665–660.

The references to insulin resistance and its relationship to obesity and other diseases can be found in:

Pawson, I.G., R. Martorell, and F.E. Mendoza. "Prevalence of Overweight and Obesity in U.S. Hispanic Populations." *American Journal of Clinical Nutrition* 53 (1991): 1522S–1528S.

Modan, M., H. Halkin, S. Almog, et al. "Hyperinsulinemia: A Link Between Hypertension, Obesity, and Glucose Intolerance." *Journal of Clinical Investigations* 15 (1985): 431–440.

The reference to collecting fat around the middle can be found in: Atkins, R.C., *Dr. Atkins' New Diet Revolution.* New York: Avon Books, 1992.

CHAPTER 19

The reference to nonepinephrine and other catecholamines and their effect on blood pressure can be found in:

"National Heart, Lung, and Blood Institute Update on Task Force Report on High Blood Pressure in Children and Adolescents." *American Family Physician* 55, no. 6 (1997): 2340–2345.

Gidding, S.S., et al. "The Committee on Atherosclerosis and Hypertension in the Young of the Council on Cardiovascular Disease in the Young and the Nutrition Committee: Understanding Obesity in Youth." *Circulation* 94 (1996): 3383–3387.

CHAPTER 20

The reference to cholesterol problems beginning in childhood can be found in: McGill, H.C., Jr., A. McMahan, et al., "Relation of glycohemoglobin and adiposity to atherosclerosis in youth." *Arteriosclerosis Thrombosis Vascular Biology* 15 (1995): 431–440.

The reference to problems with damaged arteries beginning as early as six can be found in: Worcester, S., "Smoking, Poor Cholesterol Damage Teens' Arteries." *Internal Medicine News* (April 1, 1997): 61.

The reference to an update on cardiovascular disease in children can be found in: "National Heart, Lung, and Blood Institute Update on Task Force Report on High Blood Pressure in Children and Adolescents." *American Family Physician* 55, no. 6 (1997): 2340–2345.

CHAPTER 21

The reference to favorable responses with antifungal medication on the treatment of learning disabilities can be found in:

Acta Dermatologica Venerology 186 (1994): 149–150.

Shaw, W., et al. "Abnormal Urine Organic Acids Associated with Fungal Metabolism in Urine Samples of Children with Autism: Preliminary Results of a Clinical Trial with Anti-fungal Drugs." The Proceedings Meeting of the Autism Society of America, 1995.

CHAPTER 22

The reference to childhood food allergies can be found in: Anderson, J., "Milk, Eggs, and Peanuts: Food Allergies in Children." *American Family Physician* 56, no. 5 (1997): 1365–1374.

CHAPTER 24

The reference to the increased incidence of colds in children who attend day care can be found in: Cordell, R.L., S.L. Solomon, and C.M. Hale, "Exclusion of Mildly Ill Children from Out-of-Home Child Care Facilities." *Infectious Medicine* 13, no. 41 (1996): 45–48.

The reference to the number of respiratory infections a child will get can be found in: Green, M., *Pediatric Diagnosis: Interpretation of Symptoms and Signs in Infants, Children, and Adolescents,* 5th ed., 385–392, Philadelphia, PA: WB Saunders Co., 1991.

The reference to the increased number of prescriptions issued can be found in: See Chapter 17 references.

The reference to antibiotic use and its relationship to otitis media can be found in: Gonzales, R. and M. Sande, "What Will It Take to Stop Physician's from Prescribing Antibiotics in Acute Otitis Media?" *Lancet* 345 (1995): 665–666.

The reference to ear infections and hyperactive children can be found in: Hagerman, R.J., and M.A. Falkenstein, "An Association Between Recurrent Otitis Media in Infancy and Later Hyperactivity." *Clinical Pediatrics* 26, no. 5 (1987).

CHAPTER 25

The reference to the percentage of school-age children diagnosed with ADD can be found in: Rasbury, W.C., "Attention Deficit Disorder: An Overview." *Henry Ford Hospital Medical Journal* 36, no. 4 (1988): 212–216.

The references to the diagnostic criteria for ADD can be found in: American Psychiatric Association, *Diagnostic and Statistical Manual of Mental Disorders,* 4th ed. Washington, D.C.: American Psychiatric Association, 1994.

The reference to the increase in Ritalin prescriptions can be found in: Safer, D.J., and J.M. Krager, "Trends in the Medication Treatment of Hyperactive School Children." *Clinical Pediatrics.* Philadelphia, PA. 22, no. 7 (1983): 500–504.

The reference to non-ADD children being given stimulant drugs can be found in: Rapoport, J.L., M.S. Buchsbaum, et al., "Dextroamphetamine: Its Cognitive and Behavioral Effects in Normal and Hyperactive Boys and Normal Men." *Archives of General Psychiatry* 37, no. 8 (1980): 933–943.

The reference to lead levels and their relationship to children with ADD can be found in: Gittelman, R., and B. Eskenazi, "Lead and Hyperactivity Revisited: An Investigation of Non-Disadvantaged Children." *Archives of General Psychiatry* 40 (1983): 827–833.

CHAPTER 26

The reference to long-term weight maintenance in children can be found in:

Leibel, R., and J. Hirsch, "Diminished Energy Requirements in Reduced Obese Patients." *Metabolism* 33 (1984): 164–170.

Lloyd, J., O. Wolff, and W. Whelan, "Childhood Obesity: A Long-Term Study of Height and Weight." *British Medical Journal* 2 (1961): 145–148.

CHAPTER 28

The reference to energy expenditure by overweight boys after eating can be found in: Blaak, E.E., K.R. Westerterp, et al., "Total Energy Expenditure and Spontaneous Activity in Relation to Training in Obese Boys." *American Journal of Clinical Nutrition* 55 (1992): 777–782.

The references to metabolism and the obese child can be found in:

Garrow, J.S. "Exercise, Diet, and Thermogenesis." In *Nutrition and Exercise,* edited by M. Winick. New York: John Wiley & Sons, Inc. 1986.

Maffeis, C., et al. "Meal Induced Thermogenesis in Obese Children with or without Familial History of Obesity." *European Journal of Pediatrics* 152 (1993): 128–131.

Zwiauer, K.F., et al. "Resting Metabolic Rate in Obese Children before, during and after Weight Loss." *International Journal of Obesity Related Metabolic Disorders* 16 (1992): 11–16.

Index

acetyl-l-tyrosine, 197
acne, 165, 173–74
ADD. *See* attention deficit disorder
additives, 94, 103
adolescents. *See* teenagers
alcohol avoidance, 114, 134
allergies and food sensitivities,
    138–39, 175–79
  behavior problems and, 20, 40
  to cow's milk, 101, 102, 177
  differentiated, 177–78
  to wheat, 68, 72, 120–21, 138, 177,
    178, 181
  yeast and, 138, 165–66
  See also asthma; sinusitis
amaranth, 68, 72, 120
amphetamine, 194, 196
antibiotics, overprescription of, 76,
    141–42, 162, 164, 165–66, 167, 172,
    178–79, 182, 186, 187, 189–90
antifungal medications, 172–73
antioxidants, 62, 96, 158, 181, 205–6
artichoke flour, 124
artificial sweeteners, 47–48, 103, 256
aspartame, 47, 48, 256
asthma, 40, 65, 72, 76, 138–39, 163,
    165, 180–85
attention deficit disorder, 141, 191–98
  gluten and, 72
  sugar and, 20, 40, 192
  treatments, 57, 196–98
  yeast and, 166

balance, 82, 93
behavior problems, 20, 31–32, 40
    (*see also* attention deficit disorder)
berries, 40, 43, 125
beta-carotene, 183, 184, 188, 206
beverages, 99–103 (*see also* individual
    choices)
bioflavonoids, 40, 188
blood sugar level
  balance, 79, 93, 144

diabetes and, 146–47
  glucose tolerance test, 32–34, 76
body mass index (BMI)
  formula, 76–77
  target by age group, 105, 106, 110,
    112, 114, 115
boron, 137
buckwheat, 68, 72, 120
butter, 56, 99, 126

caffeine avoidance, 39, 101, 102, 134
calcium, 99, 102, 202–3, 205
calories, 55–56, 90
camp, 216–17
cancer, 61, 67, 94
candida albicans. See yeast
canola oil, 56, 60
caprylic acid, 137, 170, 171, 181
carbohydrates, 65–72
  balance, 79, 82, 97, 106–7, 115, 123
  as blood sugar stabilizers, 79
  caveats and requirements, 97–99
  complex, 36, 97–99
  gram counter, 118–19
  "kid friendly," 117–19
  low-/high-content vegetables, 98
  simple, 36, 66–67, 68, 134
  sugars as, 36–37, 68, 97
  types of, 68
  as weight-loss busters, 103
catsup, 99, 217
cereals, list of whole grain vs. refined,
    71
CHAOS (Syndrome X related disor-
    ders), 150
cheese, 96, 119, 167, 202, 203
childhood obesity. *See* overweight child
cholesterol, 60–61, 84, 95, 150, 152,
    153–60
chromium, 206
citrus bioflavonoids, 188
coconut oil, 59
co-enzyme Q10, 219

comfort foods, 141
common cold, 178, 186, 187, 188–89
complex carbohydrates. *See* carbohydrates
condiments, 99
corn oil, 60, 62–63
corn syrup. *See* high fructose corn syrup
corticosteroids, 151–52
cow's milk. *See* milk
cyclamates, 47
cytotoxic food test, 76, 183

dairy products, 85, 96, 99, 126 (*see also* cheese; milk)
decaffeinated products, 101
desserts, 99, 119, 275–78
diabetes, 67, 143–47, 152
dietary habits
  establishing new, 93
  food as weapon, 154, 211
  hints for successful, 127–34, 212
  ignoring "odd," 128–29, 212
  as learned behavior, 133
  menus and recipes, 243–78
  portion control, 83, 130, 131–32, 134, 243
  problem situations, 213–17
  setting good example, 129, 141, 208–9
  variety in, 28
dieting. *See* weight-loss diet
diet pills, 15–16
diet soda, 102
disaccharides, 36
dyslipidemia, 150

earaches, 162, 165, 166, 187–88
eating patterns. *See* dietary habits
echinacea, 188
eczema, 185
eggs
  allergy, 177
  dietary caveats and requirements, 96
  organic, 84
  yolk, 95

egg substitutes, 96
eiconsanoids, 55
elderberry, 188
ephedra, 183–84
essential fatty acids, 56–57
evening primrose oil, 56, 58–59
exercise, 134, 218, 223–40
  aerobic benefits, 229–30
  by age group, 236–40
  as fun activity, 232–34
  injury avoidance, 235

fast food, 90, 140, 149, 157
fat cells, 27, 42
fat-enabling culture, 14–15
fats, dietary, 50–64
  advantages, 91
  calories and, 55–56
  cholesterol and, 158
  energy storage, 54, 90
  fish caveats, 95
  good/bad/ugly, 58–63, 96
  health role, 52–55
  meat caveats, 95, 157
  myths about, 50–52
  triglycerides and, 160
fatty acids, 55–57, 84
fen-phen, 16
fiber, 43, 68, 97, 99
fish, 57, 85–86
  dietary caveats and requirements, 95
"five-minute warning," 129–30
flaxseed oil, 56, 58
flu, 188, 189
folic acid, 137, 188, 200, 205
food cravings, 130, 207
food diary, 80–81, 154, 210, 217
Food Guide Pyramid, U.S.D.A., 88–90
food habits. *See* dietary habits
food sensitivities. *See* allergies and food sensitivities
free radicals, 62, 64, 96, 206
fructose, 37–40, 67
fruit juice caveats, 18, 19, 32, 38, 40, 103, 125, 134, 167

fruits
  carbohydrate grams, 118
  caveats, 18-19, 37, 124–25
  highest/lowest glycemic indexes,
    40, 43, 125
  as weight-loss buster, 103

GABA, 197
galactose, 37
garlic, 170, 176, 179, 181, 188
gelatin, sugar-free, 99, 256
genestein, 137
genetics, obesity relationship, 26–27
ginkgo biloba, 219
GLA, 154
glucagon, 34
glucose, 37, 41
glucose tolerance test, 32–34, 76, 153,
  192
gluten, 72, 98, 120, 124, 139, 178, 184
glycemic index, 37
  highest/lowest fruits and vegetables,
    40, 43, 125
  list of common foods, 42
  vs. glycemic load, 41
golf, 238–39
grains
  carbohydrate grams, 119
  chart of whole vs. refined, 69
  in forever diet, 124
  health caveats, 98
  phase one requirements, 98
  phase two allowances, 120–21
  sensitivities, 68, 72, 120–21, 177,
    178, 180–81, 184
  wheat alternatives, 68–70, 72, 98
  whole as better, 68–71, 97, 124
green leafy vegetables, 98, 99, 102,
  125, 203

health-consciousness, 137–240
  six to eight-year olds, 108
  nine to twelve-year-olds, 112
  teenagers, 116
heart disease, 67, 150, 152, 154, 200
  risk determination, 155–61

herbal decaffeinated teas, 100, 102
heritability, obesity, 26–27
high blood pressure. *See* hypertension
high fructose corn syrup, 38, 39–40
homocysteine, 156, 200
homogenization, 63–64, 101
honey, 38
hormones, 55, 151–52
household chores, 238
hydrogenation, 60, 61–63, 87, 96
hyperactivity. *See* attention deficit
  disorder
hyperplastic obesity, 27
hypertension, 148–52, 229–30
hypertrophic obesity, 27
hypoglycemia, 33, 34–35, 144, 152

immune system, 57, 72, 177, 230
inositol, 197
insulin, 33, 34, 37, 41–42, 92, 97, 98,
  160, 206
  diabetes and, 144–47
  Syndrome X and, 150–51

kamut, 68
kasha, 68, 120
kava-kava, 197
ketosis, 114

label reading, 61, 66–67, 101, 134
L-carnitine, 218
lead, 196
"leaky-gut" syndrome, 177
lecithin, 95, 154, 157
legumes, 121
lemon juice, 99
L-glutamine, 207
linoleic acid, 56
linolenic acid, 56
lipid blood profile, 150
lobbyists, 53–54
low-fat diet myths, 51–54, 64, 201
"low-fat" foods, 15, 44, 66, 87, 96, 255

macronutrients, 29–30
magnesium, 102, 188, 205

manganese, 179
margarine, 60–61, 126
mayonnaise, 99, 167
mealtime, 130–32, 134, 212
  menus and recipes, 243–78
meats
  caveats and requirements, 94, 103, 157
  organically raised, 84–85
  processed, 94, 103, 244
  saturated fats in, 56
melons, 40, 43, 125
menstrual cycle, 137–38, 205
menus, 243–54
mercury contamination, 86
metabolism, 29–30, 39, 90
  chromium as key nutrient, 206
  dietary balance of, 82, 88, 91, 97–98, 218
  exercise and, 218
  ketosis and, 114
  reregulation, 92
  sugar problems, 19
  ways to increase, 218–29
milk
  allergy, 102, 177
  carbohydrate grams, 119
  caveats and requirements, 68, 101–2, 103, 134, 139
  homogenized, 63–64, 102
  mother's vs. cow's, 29
  organic, 85
  as overrated calcium source, 202, 203
millet, 68, 72, 120
monosaccharides, 36
monosodium glutamate (MSG), 94, 103
monounsaturated fats, 51, 54, 55–56
multivitamins, 206
mushrooms, 167
mustard, 99, 167
mycocidin, 137

Next Generation Diet, 75–134, 147
  as forever diet, 123–24

nutritional supplements, 199–207, 218–19
  success tips, 127–33
Next Generation Food Pyramid, 88–90
nine to twelve-year-olds
  diet plan, 109–12, 209–10, 211
  exercise, 237–38
nitrates and nitrites, 94, 103, 244
"no sugar added" products, 67
NutraSweet, 48
nutritional supplements, 199–207
  for acne, 174
  for allergies, 176, 179
  for asthma, 181, 183, 184
  for attention deficit disorder, 197, 198
  for blood sugar control, 147
  calcium as, 102
  for colds, sore throats, and earaches, 188, 189
  for elevated cholesterol, 154, 157
  for menstrual irregularity, 137
  for Syndrome X, 149–50, 152
  for weight control, 218–19
  for yeast control, 170–71
nuts and seeds, 119, 120, 124
Nystatin, 172

oats, 120, 124
obesity. See overweight child
oils, 59–60, 62–63, 87, 96
olive oil, 56, 58, 63, 99
omega-3 fatty acids, 56–57, 59–60, 84, 154, 155–56, 157, 176, 185, 197, 198
omega-6 fatty acids, 56–57, 59–60, 84, 154, 185, 198
orange juice, 40
oranges, 43
organic foods, 83–84, 134, 244
overeating, portion control vs., 83
overweight child
  body mass index test, 76–77
  diabetes risk, 144–46
  early signs, 17
  family attitudes and, 25–28

fruit juice link, 103
heritability factor, 26–27
number of fat cells vs. amount of fat
  per cell, 27
puberty developmental problems,
  138
reasons for, 17–18
self-esteem and, 21–23, 128
successful dieting tips, 128–33
See also weight-loss diet
oxidation, 96

palm oil, 59
pancreas, 34, 37
pantethine, 154, 157
parties, 213–14
pastas, 70, 124
pasteurization, 101
peanut oil, 59–60
phagocytosis, 72
phosphatidyl sereine, 197
phosphorous, 102, 202
picky eaters, 211–12
plums, 40, 43, 125
polyunsaturated fats, 51, 54, 56–57
portion control, 83, 94, 130, 131–32,
  134, 243
potato chips (baked), 39
potatoes (white and sweet), 98, 167
poultry, 86, 95
preschooler exercise, 236
probiotics, 171–72, 181
processed foods, 61, 62–63, 64, 66
  American cheese caveat, 96
  avoidance of, 86–87, 134, 172
  high sugar content, 44, 66, 86–87
  luncheon meats, 94, 103, 244
  milk, 101
  as weight-loss busters, 103
prostaglandins, 55
proteins
  child's needs, 30
  dietary advantages, 91
  dietary balance, 79, 82, 115, 123
  Next Generation Diet phase I, 93–96
  organic sources, 84–85

psyche, balanced, 93
puberty, 138
pyramid. *See* Food Pyramid

quercetin, 176, 179, 184, 188
quinoa, 70, 72, 120

rancidity, 61–62
recipes, 255–78
recommended daily allowances
  (RDAs), 202
rice, 72
rice milk, 101, 102
Ritalin, 192, 193–94, 196
rutin, 188
rye, 120, 124

saccharin, safety of, 47, 255, 256
safflower oil, 60
St. John's wort, 197
salicylates, 196–97
salt, 87
saturated fats, 51, 54, 56
school day eating, 18, 214–15
selenium, 188
self-esteem, 21–25, 128, 232
seltzer, 256
serotonin, 197
sesame oil, 60
sinusitis, 189–90
six to eight-year-olds
  diet plan, 104–8, 209
  exercise, 237–38
snack foods, 39, 215–16
soda (soft drinks), 18, 19, 37, 38, 39
  fruit juice similarity, 19, 125
  restrictions, 100, 102, 134
  type permitted, 100
sodium. *See* salt
sore throat, 188–89
soybean oil, 60, 62–63
soy flour, 98
soy milk, 101, 102, 119
spelt, 70
starch, 68, 98
stearic acid, 56

stevia, 48–49, 255–56
strep throat, 188–89
sucrose, 38
sugar, 31–49
    artificial sweeteners vs., 47–48
    in complex carbohydrates, 97
    content in specific foods, 37–39, 42,
        44–46
    cravings, 207
    dietary balance, 123, 144
    diet elimination, 79, 134, 172
    in fruits and fruit juice, 18, 19, 32,
        38, 125
    hidden, 38–39, 66–67, 86–87, 94,
        217–18
    in milk, 102
    mood effects, 75
    mouthfeel quality, 44, 96
    per capita U.S. consumption, 37
    poor health effects, 34–35, 66, 72,
        139, 144
    in processed meats, 94
    as reward, 19–20
    as simple carbohydrate, 68
    as weight-loss buster, 103
    See also glucose tolerance test;
        glycemic index
sweeteners. See artificial sweeteners
sweets
    carbohydrate grams, 119
    as reward, 19–20
    See also sugar
Syndrome X, 148–52

teas, 100, 101, 102
teenagers
    diet plan, 113–16, 132, 210–11
    exercise plan, 239–40
teff, 70, 120
television viewing, 225
tempeh, 121
theophylline, 184
thyroid gland, 29
tofu, 121
trans fatty acids, 51, 60, 61, 96
transition diet

six to eight-year olds, 106–8
    nine to twelve-year-olds, 110–12
    teenagers, 114–15
    from yeast-free diet, 168–69
triglycerides, 52, 150, 155, 157, 159–60

vegetable juices, 125
vegetables, 18–19, 120, 206
    carbohydrate grams, 118
    caveats and requirements, 98, 167
    dietary balance, 115
    glycemic index, 42, 43
    green leafy, 98, 99, 102, 125, 203
video exercise tapes, 239
vinegars, 99, 167, 217
vitamin A, 176, 179, 184
vitamin B complex, 97, 198
vitamin C, 19, 29, 62, 158, 176, 179,
    181, 183, 188, 206
vitamin D_3, 102, 205
vitamin E, 62, 97, 158, 183, 206
vitamins, fat-soluble, 55
vitamin supplements, 201–2

water, 99–100, 102, 256
weight, ideal, 77
weight-loss diet
    six to eight-year-olds, 105
    nine to twelve-year-olds, 110
    busters, 99, 103
    nutritional supplements, 201–2,
        206–7
    steps to take if no weight loss,
        217–18
    teenagers, 113
wheat germ, 70
wheat sensitivity, 68, 72, 120–21, 138,
    177, 178, 181

yeast, 162–74, 176–77
yeast-free diet, 138, 167–69, 173–74,
    181, 183, 185
yeast infection, 162, 165–67, 190
yogurt, 126, 203

zinc, 188, 198